Sweet and Slick

The Impact of Excessive Sugar and
Processed Oils on Our Health

By
Well-Being Publishing

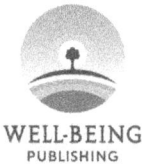

Sweet and Slick

The Impact of Excessive Sugar and
Processed Oils on Our Health

Table of Contents

Understanding the Sweetness and Slipperiness of Modern Diets

In today's world, the adage "you are what you eat" takes on a profound significance. As we navigate the aisles of our local supermarkets, we're often bombarded with an overwhelming variety of food choices, many of which are laden with sugars and processed fats. These ingredients, so seamlessly integrated into our diets, wield a substantial influence on our health. Yet, understanding their true impact can often feel like untangling a complex web. In this introduction, we aim to unravel the entwined relationships between our dietary choices and our well-being, guiding you toward a more informed and health-conscious lifestyle.

Modern diets are characterized by their convenience and palatability, a trend driven by the food industry's relentless pursuit of profit and efficiency. However, the hidden costs to our health are becoming increasingly undeniable. The ubiquity of sugars and processed oils in our food has been linked to an array of chronic health conditions, from obesity and diabetes to heart disease and inflammation (Lustig, 2013). Understanding these links is crucial for anyone looking to make healthier dietary choices.

Human history illuminates our evolving relationship with food. Ancient diets were composed mainly of whole, unprocessed foods, rich in natural fats and scarce in refined sugars. Fast forward to the 20th century, and we witness an industrial revolution in our food supply. Mass production techniques made sugar and vegetable oils cheap and abundant, and their integration into the food system was nothing

1

short of revolutionary (Moss, 2013). This shift not only changed the way food tasted but also how it affected our bodies.

The convenience of modern diets often comes at the expense of nutritional quality. Processed foods, laden with "hidden" sugars and unhealthy fats, lure us with their immediate gratification. Yet, the long-term impact on our health can be detrimental. Studies indicate that high consumption of added sugars contributes to insulin resistance, a precursor to both Type 2 diabetes and a host of metabolic disorders (Hu & Malik, 2010). Likewise, the role of trans fats and hydrogenated oils in promoting inflammation and cardiovascular diseases has been well documented (Mozaffarian et al., 2010).

Given these insights, it's natural to wonder how we can navigate this landscape more wisely. The first step is education—recognizing the ingredients that do our bodies harm and understanding the science behind their effects. For instance, sugars act not only as sweeteners but also as preservatives, thickeners, and fermenting agents in a wide array of products. Their various forms—from glucose and sucrose to high-fructose corn syrup—interact differently with our metabolism and hormones, often exacerbating health issues like obesity and systemic inflammation (Stanhope, 2012).

Similarly, not all fats are created equal. While natural fats from whole foods can be beneficial, the processed oils ubiquitous in fast food and ready-to-eat meals often contain trans fats. These fats are chemically altered to enhance shelf life but at the expense of our cardiovascular health. They can raise LDL ("bad") cholesterol levels while lowering HDL ("good") cholesterol, a combination that increases the risk of heart disease (Willett, 2012).

Transforming our approach to diet means more than just eliminating certain ingredients. It's about reconceptualizing what we consider to be "food." Instead of seeing food as mere fuel, we should view it as a multifaceted entity that influences every aspect of our health. Embracing whole foods—vegetables, fruits, whole grains, and natural proteins—can provide the nutrients our bodies need to thrive while avoiding the pitfalls associated with processed sugars and oils.

The journey toward a healthier diet is a gradual process, filled with small but impactful changes. It begins with informed choices, progressing through the conscious reduction of processed foods, and culminates in a balanced, whole-food-centric diet. The benefits of making these changes can be profound, not just for individual health, but for the well-being of our communities and the sustainability of our environment.

This book aims to be your companion on this journey, providing you with the knowledge and tools to make better dietary choices. We will delve into the history and science of sugars and oils, highlight their roles and risks, and offer practical guidance for integrating healthier alternatives into your daily routine. Whether you're a health-conscious individual, a parent looking to set a better example for your children, a patient managing a chronic condition, or a healthcare professional seeking to deepen your understanding, the insights and strategies presented here are geared to empower you.

Real change starts with awareness and intention. By taking the time to understand the sweetness and slipperiness of our modern diets, we're better positioned to make choices that benefit our long-term health. The goal is not just to survive, but to thrive—living vibrant, energetic lives through conscious, informed eating.

In the chapters that follow, we'll explore these topics in depth, separating myth from fact and providing clear, actionable advice. We'll dissect the history of dietary changes, classify different types of sugars and fats, examine their effects on our health, and offer practical strategies for everyday life. By the end of this book, you'll be armed with the knowledge to make smarter choices and the inspiration to follow through with lasting lifestyle changes.

Our collective health depends on the choices we make today. Understanding the complexities of sugar and processed oils is the first step toward reclaiming our well-being. Let's embark on this journey together, informed and empowered to navigate the sweetness and slipperiness of modern diets with wisdom and care.

Chapter 1:
The History of Sugar
and Processed Oils

The journey of sugar and processed oils has profoundly shaped our dietary landscape, transitioning from rare, natural sources in ancient times to ubiquitous elements in modern diets. Originally, sugar was a luxury, derived from sugar cane introduced by Middle Eastern and North African traders to Europe (Kiple & Ornelas, 2000). Over centuries, with the advent of sugar beets and large-scale production methods, sugar became widely accessible, embedding itself into daily consumption patterns and contributing to numerous health issues (Lustig et al., 2012). In parallel, the rise of processed oils, particularly from the late 19th century, revolutionized cooking and food preservation. The industrial extraction of vegetable oils shifted dietary fats from traditional animal sources to manufactured ones like margarine, often laden with trans fats (Teicholz, 2014). This shift, largely driven by market forces and technological innovations, overlooked the long-term health implications, connecting these dietary changes to the rising incidence of chronic diseases (Mozaffarian & Clarke, 2009). Understanding the historical context of these transformations is crucial for making informed, healthier dietary choices today.

From Antiquity to Modern Times: The Evolution of Sweeteners traces the fascinating journey of sweeteners from their early beginnings to their current, complex role in our diets today. The story starts in the ancient world.

In ancient civilizations, sweetness wasn't as ubiquitous as it is now. Honey was among the earliest known sweeteners, documented in Egyptian hieroglyphs dating back to 2400 BCE. Known as "the nectar of the gods," honey was not only a sweet treat but also held medicinal properties (Barrett, 2002). Honey was later joined by date syrup in the Middle East and even maple syrup by indigenous North American tribes, demonstrating early methods for extracting natural sweetness from the environment.

Fast forward to classical antiquity, sugarcane cultivation started in India around 6,000 years ago. This sweet grass was highly revered, and its juice, obtained by crushing the cane, was a luxury item. The rest of the world started to catch on when Alexander the Great's armies brought pieces of sugar cane back from India (Kiple & Ornelas, 2000).

In medieval times, sugar's rise to prominence in Europe began. Often referred to as "white gold," it was extremely expensive and primarily used by the wealthy. This era also saw the cultivation of sugarcane spread to new territories, including the Mediterranean and Spain. The eventual colonization of the Americas in the 15th century marked the beginning of large-scale sugar production. Caribbean plantations became notorious for their productivity and for the brutal enslavement of people to meet the European demand for sugar (Mintz, 1985).

The industrial revolution brought about significant changes in the production of sweeteners. By the mid-19th century, technological advancements made sugar more affordable and accessible. Sugar beet cultivation in Europe and North America added another dimension to production. Because of these developments, sugar shifted from being a luxury to a staple. This period also witnessed the discovery of artificial sweeteners like saccharin, offering calorie-free alternatives (Yudkin,

1972). This innovation opened the doors for the production of other synthetic sweeteners such as aspartame and sucralose.

Modern times have complicated our relationship with sweetness even further. Today, sweeteners can be broadly divided into two categories: natural and artificial. Natural sweeteners include familiar options like honey, maple syrup, and agave nectar, but also feature less common ones like stevia and monk fruit. These natural sweeteners bring the advantage of having additional nutrients, and some have a lower glycemic index compared to table sugar. For example, stevia, derived from the leaves of the Stevia rebaudiana plant, has become popular for its zero-calorie content and lack of impact on blood sugar levels (Goyal et al., 2010).

Artificial sweeteners, once hailed as miracle substitutes, have found themselves at the center of health debates. Critics argue that some can disrupt metabolism and contribute to weight gain. On the other hand, proponents highlight the advantages such as caloric reduction and dental health benefits (Swithers, 2013). However, the scientific consensus about their long-term safety remains divided.

As our understanding of nutrition evolves, we've also seen a push towards understanding the impact of high-fructose corn syrup (HFCS), an omnipresent ingredient in sodas and processed foods. With a composition that allows it to deliver intense sweetness, HFCS has been linked to various health issues, including obesity and metabolic syndrome (Bray et al., 2004). Even though it was initially introduced as a cost-effective alternative to cane sugar, the health costs associated with its consumption have sparked a reconsideration of its widespread use.

The evolution of sweeteners has also paralleled advances in food science. Today, we see the advent of hybrid products combining artificial and natural elements to create a balance between taste and health benefits. Products like erythritol-based sweeteners and allulose are gaining popularity for their minimal impact on blood sugar levels and closer mimicry of sucrose's taste profile.

It's crucial to recognize that while sweeteners have evolved, so have our tastes and consumption habits. The modern diet has made sugar and sweeteners a central feature, often leading to overconsumption. For instance, the average American now consumes over 17 teaspoons of added sugar per day, far exceeding the American Heart Association's recommendations (AHA, 2019).

Ironically, the solutions to some of these modern dietary problems may lie in looking back at history. Reintegrating natural sweeteners into our diets, albeit in moderation, can be a step towards better health. Understanding historical patterns of sweetener use can provide meaningful insights and guide more informed decisions.

As you continue reading this book, you'll come across critiques and discussions of other processed ingredients that shape our current dietary landscape. For now, let's retain a nuanced view of sweeteners. By blending historical context with scientific research, we can make better choices that favor both our palates and our health.

In sum, sweeteners have come a long way from their primitive origins. Their evolution reveals much about human ingenuity, economic development, and the adaptive nature of our diets. As we move forward, understanding this history can help steer us toward healthier choices and more sustainable consumption patterns.

Vegetable Oils and Margarine: The Rise of Processed Fats have a significant impact on our dietary landscape, and their journey from obscurity to pantry staples warrants a closer look. They may seem ubiquitous now, but the origin and proliferation of vegetable oils and margarine are stories of industrial innovation, marketing magic, and a complex dance with health science. This examination unveils the shifts in our health narratives and the transformations in our everyday lives.

In the late 19th and early 20th centuries, the advent of industrial processing techniques revolutionized food production. The introduction of hydrogenation, which solidifies liquid oils, allowed for the mass production of margarine and shortening from plant-based oils. Margarine, originally designed as a substitute for butter, became increasingly popular during World War II when butter was scarce. By the mid-20th century, vegetable oils derived from corn, soybean, and cottonseed plants became staple ingredients in many households due to their affordability and versatility (Ghosh et al., 2021).

The initial appeal of these oils lay in their cost-effectiveness and stability. Unlike animal fats, vegetable oils could be stored for longer periods without becoming rancid. This made them an attractive option for both home cooks and food manufacturers striving for longer shelf-life products. However, the processing methods required to make these oils stable often involve high temperatures and chemical solvents, which can strip the oils of their natural antioxidants and nutrients (Mozaffarian, 2006).

Health authorities and food industries further propelled the rise of vegetable oils and margarine by promoting them as healthier alternatives to saturated animal fats. During the cholesterol frenzy of the 1970s and 1980s, saturated fats found in butter, lard, and tropical oils were vilified for their role in raising "bad" LDL cholesterol. This led to a widespread adoption of polyunsaturated fats, particularly linoleic acid from vegetable oils, believed to lower cardiovascular risks (Keys et al., 1984). However, emerging research has begun to question these once-universal recommendations.

The crux of the issue lies in the oxidative instability of polyunsaturated fatty acids (PUFAs). While they can indeed lower LDL cholesterol, PUFAs are highly susceptible to oxidation, a process that produces reactive oxygen species capable of damaging cells and promoting inflammation. Chronic inflammation is now recognized as a key driver of many chronic diseases, including heart disease, cancer, and neurodegenerative disorders (Simopoulos, 2002). Thus, the initial promise of vegetable oils as heart-healthy alternatives is now subject to ongoing scientific scrutiny (Ramsden et al., 2013).

Add to this the problem of trans fats, which are created during the partial hydrogenation process to solidify vegetable oils. Trans fats have been unequivocally linked to adverse health outcomes, including increased risk of coronary artery disease, by raising LDL cholesterol and lowering "good" HDL cholesterol (Mozaffarian et al., 2006). The harmful effects of trans fats led to regulatory actions worldwide, including the U.S. FDA's decision to eliminate trans fats from the food supply in June 2018. Yet, the legacy of decades of trans fat consumption remains a public health concern.

So, where do we stand now? Our understanding of dietary fats has evolved, with a growing appreciation for the complexities of different fat types and their respective health impacts. Today, many nutrition experts advocate for a return to whole, minimally processed fats found in nature, such as extra virgin olive oil, avocado, nuts, and seeds. These sources provide a valuable mix of monounsaturated and natural polyunsaturated fats, along with essential nutrients (Harvard T.H. Chan School of Public Health, n.d.).

In an increasingly health-conscious world, consumers are becoming more discerning. The once-unquestioned dominance of vegetable oils and margarine faces challenges from an informed public seeking to prioritize health over convenience. This shift is evident in the growing popularity of products such as grass-fed butter, ghee, and coconut oil, all of which boast nutrient profiles free from the oxidative stress associated with heavily processed oils.

Yet, the transformation from processed fats to healthier alternatives isn't just about personal choices. It's also about systemic changes in food production and regulatory policies. Encouraging transparency in labeling, supporting sustainable farming practices, and educating communities about the long-term effects of dietary fats are essential steps towards healthier eating habits (Nestle, 2013).

The rise of processed fats in the form of vegetable oils and margarine represents a fascinating, if cautionary, chapter in our culinary history. As with any nutritional trend, it's crucial to balance innovative convenience with empirical evidence and thoughtful consumption. Understanding the journey of these fats—from their industrial beginnings to their current status—empowers us to make well-informed dietary decisions. The pursuit of health is not just about eliminating or avoiding specific ingredients but about cultivating a comprehensive, nuanced approach to nutrition.

In conclusion, while vegetable oils and margarine have played pivotal roles in modern diets, their health implications necessitate a re-evaluation. With an eye on evolving scientific insights and a commitment to well-being, we can navigate our dietary choices more wisely. By embracing both tradition and innovation, we can nourish ourselves and future generations more holistically and sustainably.

For those interested in an in-depth journey through the complex landscape of dietary fats, the preceding sections provide a robust framework, exploring various facets of fats and oils in our diets. Recognizing the significance of these discussions, your feedback and reflections are incredibly valuable to us. Please consider sharing your thoughts online to help others on their path to nutritional enlightenment.

Chapter 2:
Sugar Defined: Types and
Their Roles in Food

Understanding the various types of sugar is essential for making informed dietary choices. Sugars, essentially carbohydrates, can be classified into natural and added categories, each playing distinct roles in our food. Natural sugars, such as those found in fruits (fructose) and dairy products (lactose), are accompanied by fibers, vitamins, and minerals that aid in digestion and overall health. Added sugars, on the other hand, such as sucrose and high-fructose corn syrup, are commonly incorporated into processed foods and beverages to enhance flavor, texture, and shelf life but offer no nutritional benefits (Johnson et al., 2009). The widespread use of added sugars has been linked to various health risks, including obesity, diabetes, and heart disease (Malik et al., 2010). Therefore, it's crucial to distinguish between these types of sugars and understand their roles and implications to make smarter dietary decisions.

Natural vs. Added Sugars: What's the Difference? can be the turning point in making smarter dietary choices for us and our loved ones. By understanding the distinction between these two, we empower ourselves to take control of our health and well-being. Natural sugars and added sugars may seem alike, but they are worlds apart both in terms of their sources and their effects on our bodies.

Natural sugars are intrinsic to whole foods. Found in fruits, vegetables, and dairy products, these sugars are accompanied by essential nutrients such as vitamins, minerals, and fiber. Think of the sweetness you get from biting into an apple or savoring a ripe banana. The presence of these nutrients helps in the gradual absorption of sugar, preventing sudden spikes in blood glucose levels (Livesey, 2009). Moreover, the fiber content in fruit slows down digestion, making us feel full longer and aiding digestive health (Slavin, 2005).

On the other hand, added sugars are those that aren't inherently part of the food. They're inserted during the processing or preparation stages. Common sources include sweetened beverages, candies, baked goods, and desserts. Unfortunately, these sugars contribute to empty calories—calories devoid of nutritional value (Johnson et al., 2009). When sugars are added without accompanying nutrients, they lead to rapid glucose absorption, spiking blood sugar levels and often consequential energy crashes, not to mention long-term health issues like obesity, diabetes, and heart disease.

It's important to delineate the extent of their impact. For instance, consider high-fructose corn syrup (HFCS), one of the most notorious added sugars. Widely used in the food industry due to its cost-effectiveness and sweeter taste, HFCS has been linked with various metabolic disorders. Studies suggest that added fructose, such as that found in HFCS, can lead to increased fat production in the liver and greater insulin resistance (Stanhope et al., 2012). Conversely, the natural fructose in fruits is not only less concentrated but is also mitigated by fiber and antioxidants, making it less harmful.

To put it simply, the context in which sugar is consumed matters. A soda and an orange both contain sugar, but the former is filled with added sugars while the latter is rich in natural sugars along with fiber, vitamin C, and other nutrients. One spikes your blood sugar almost immediately, while the other provides a steady stream of energy over a longer period.

Another perspective is the energy and satiety issue. Foods with natural sugars generally offer satiety and prolonged energy. In contrast, added sugars often lead to more cravings and the consumption of extra calories. Therefore, understanding these differences helps guide not only our choices but also our behaviors towards food—helping us move from high-sugar, low-nutrient foods to nutritionally rich options.

The path to reduced sugar intake starts with awareness and reading labels carefully. With added sugars lurking in unexpected places like savory dressings and processed meats, it's critical to check ingredient lists and nutritional panels. Terms like "sucrose," "corn syrup," "fruit juice concentrates," and "molasses" are indicators of added sugars (USDA, 2021). Therefore, making a habit of scrutinizing food labels can be a game changer.

As we navigate through this, it's worth noting that the food industry is catching up to the demand for lower-sugar options. Many products now pride themselves on being free from added sugars or use natural sweeteners like stevia and monk fruit. While these alternatives might offer some respite, they too should be consumed in moderation. The focus should always remain on whole, unprocessed foods.

In educating the next generation, particularly our children, about the differences between natural and added sugars, we lay the foundation for lifelong healthy eating habits. Children are particularly susceptible to high sugar intake, which not only affects their physical health but also impacts cognitive function and behavioral patterns (Taras, 2005). Reduced sugar consumption can lead to better academic performances and fewer mood swings.

For the fitness enthusiasts and healthcare professionals, understanding this disparity can inform better dietary recommendations. From crafting personalized meal plans to community education on healthier eating habits, emphasizing the importance of natural sugars can yield significant health benefits. This knowledge is crucial for those managing specific health conditions like diabetes or obesity, where the type and source of sugar play a critical role in managing symptoms and overall health outcomes.

Remember, it's not about entirely cutting out sugar, but making conscious choices about the types of sugars we consume. Transitioning to a diet rich in natural sugars rather than added sugars is a step towards sustainable health. Think of it as swapping out sodas for a refreshing fruit salad, or choosing plain yogurt over flavored ones loaded with hidden sugars. These small changes can collectively bring about significant health transformations.

To wrap up, always remember that the quality of sweeteners in your diet matters just as much as the quantity. By prioritizing natural sugars and minimizing added sugars, you set the stage for better health, longevity, and overall wellness. With the arsenal of knowledge at your disposal, the power to make informed choices is in your hands. Make every bite count.

Sweeteners Unveiled: From Glucose to High-Fructose Corn Syrup Sugar, in its various forms, plays a pivotal role in our lives, often making its way into the foods we consume daily. Understanding the different types of sweeteners, from the simple glucose to the more complex high-fructose corn syrup, is vital for making informed dietary choices. Let's delve into these sweeteners and uncover their effects on our health and everyday consumption.

First, let's talk about glucose, a simple sugar and the most basic form of carbohydrate. It's found naturally in many foods, including fruits and honey. Our bodies rely on glucose as a primary source of energy, breaking down the carbohydrates we consume into this essential sugar. However, not all glucose is created equal. The glucose in whole foods is absorbed more slowly into the bloodstream due to the presence of fiber, which helps moderate blood sugar levels (Jenkins et al., 1981).

Moving up the complexity ladder, we encounter sucrose, commonly known as table sugar. Sucrose is a disaccharide composed of one molecule of glucose and one of fructose. It's found naturally in many plants but most abundantly in sugar cane and sugar beets. When consumed, the body breaks down sucrose into its component sugars, glucose and fructose, which are then absorbed into the bloodstream (Rumessen & Gudmand-Hoyer, 1986).

Fructose, often referred to as fruit sugar, is found naturally in fruits, honey, and root vegetables. It's sweeter than glucose and sucrose, making it a popular choice for sweetening foods and beverages. The metabolism of fructose is different from that of glucose; it primarily occurs in the liver, where it can be converted into glucose and stored as fat if consumed in excess. This unique metabolic pathway has raised concerns about its potential contribution to obesity and metabolic disorders when consumed in large amounts (Bray et al., 2004).

Enter high-fructose corn syrup (HFCS), a sweetener engineered to extend the shelf-life and enhance the sweetness of processed foods. HFCS is derived from corn starch and contains varying proportions of glucose and fructose. The most common form, HFCS-55, is composed of 55% fructose and 45% glucose, closely mimicking the sugar content of sucrose (White, 2008). However, HFCS has been scrutinized for potentially exacerbating the obesity epidemic and associated metabolic conditions due to its high fructose content (Stanhope et al., 2009).

The rise of HFCS in the food industry coincides with increased rates of obesity and diabetes, leading some researchers to investigate potential links. Studies have suggested that HFCS may contribute more significantly to these conditions than other forms of sugar, due to its metabolic impacts (Lustig, 2010). However, other researchers argue that when consumed in moderate amounts, HFCS is not more harmful than other sweeteners (White, 2008). The debate continues, but caution is warranted given the pervasive presence of HFCS in processed foods.

It's also essential to consider the broader context of sweetener consumption within the dietary landscape. Over the last few decades, there has been a notable increase in the consumption of processed foods laden with added sugars, including HFCS. This shift has significant implications for public health, influencing everything from weight gain and dental health to the risk of chronic diseases such as type 2 diabetes and cardiovascular issues (Malik et al., 2010).

For health-conscious individuals and families, understanding these nuances in sweetener types can empower better food choices. Opting for natural sugars found in whole fruits and minimizing the intake of foods with added sugars, especially those containing HFCS, can be an effective strategy for maintaining balanced blood sugar levels and overall health.

Given these complexities, it's crucial to approach sweetener consumption with informed caution. This involves not only scrutinizing food labels for hidden sugars (which will be further discussed in "Reading Between the Labels") but also understanding the metabolic pathways and health impacts of these sweeteners. As parents, healthcare professionals, and educators, imparting this knowledge can aid in crafting diets that prioritize whole foods and natural sweetness over processed alternatives.

In preparation for the "Online Review Request for This Book" section, we invite you to reflect on how understanding the diversity and impacts of sweeteners has influenced your dietary choices. By navigating through the intricate world of glucose, sucrose, fructose, and HFCS, are you more empowered to make healthier decisions for yourself and your loved ones?

As you continue to explore the various chapters of this book, you'll gain further insights into how these and other dietary components affect our health. We hope this information not only enlightens but motivates you to spread awareness and foster healthier eating habits within your community. Remember, every small step towards understanding and action can lead to monumental changes in your overall well-being.

Chapter 3:
The Oil Spectrum: Identifying Healthy Fats

Understanding the spectrum of fats is crucial for making informed dietary choices that promote long-term health. Saturated, monounsaturated, and polyunsaturated fats each play distinct roles in our bodies, from energy production to cellular function. While saturated fats, like those found in animal products and certain oils, have been historically debated, recent research shows they aren't the enemy we once thought (Siri-Tarino et al., 2010). Monounsaturated fats, abundant in olive oil and avocados, are celebrated for their heart-protective benefits and ability to reduce inflammation (Bhupathiraju & Hu, 2016). Polyunsaturated fats, including essential omega-3 and omega-6 fatty acids, are vital for brain function and cell growth, yet balancing these fats is key to avoiding chronic inflammation (Simopoulos, 2002). By distinguishing these fats, we empower ourselves to choose oils that nourish rather than harm, setting the path toward a healthier future.

Understanding Saturated, Monounsaturated, and Polyunsaturated Fats is a crucial aspect of navigating the complex landscape of dietary oils and their health implications. Armed with this understanding, you can make informed choices that promote long-term well-being. This section dives deep into the structures, sources, health benefits, and risks associated with these fats, helping you discern how they fit into a balanced diet.

Saturated fats are often labeled as unhealthy, primarily because they can raise low-density lipoprotein (LDL) cholesterol levels, commonly referred to as "bad" cholesterol. These fats are typically solid at room temperature and are found in animal products like butter, cheese, and fatty meats, as well as tropical oils such as coconut oil and palm oil. While excessive saturated fat intake has been linked to cardiovascular diseases (Santaren et al., 2018), the role of these fats is more nuanced. For instance, some studies have shown that not all saturated fats have the same impact on heart health. Moreover, dietary guidelines suggest that saturated fats can be part of a balanced diet when consumed in moderation (Eaton, 2019).

On the other hand, monounsaturated fats are generally celebrated for their health benefits. These fats are liquid at room temperature and are abundant in foods like olive oil, avocados, and nuts. Monounsaturated fats have been shown to improve heart health by reducing LDL cholesterol levels while maintaining or even increasing high-density lipoprotein (HDL) or "good" cholesterol (Astrup et al., 2020). This heart-healthy profile makes them a staple in the Mediterranean diet, which is lauded for its numerous health benefits, including reduced risks of cardiovascular disease and improved cognitive function.

Polyunsaturated fats, which include omega-3 and omega-6 fatty acids, are another category that offers significant health benefits. Omega-3 fatty acids, found in fish like salmon and flaxseeds, are anti-inflammatory and have been linked to heart health, reduced arthritis symptoms, and improved brain function (Simopoulos, 2016). Omega-6 fatty acids, found in vegetable oils like corn and soybean oil, also play an essential role in the body but should be consumed in balance with omega-3s to prevent potential inflammatory effects. Overconsumption of omega-6 fatty acids, especially from processed foods, has been linked to chronic inflammation and related health issues like heart disease and arthritis (Calder, 2015).

Understanding the varying roles these fats play in our health is essential for crafting a balanced diet. Each type of fat impacts our body differently, and the goal should be to optimize our intake to support overall well-being. This means incorporating a variety of healthy fats while limiting those that may pose health risks. Knowing these differences empowers you to make better dietary choices, which is increasingly essential in a world where processed foods high in unhealthy fats are ubiquitous.

So, how do you bring this knowledge into your everyday life? Start by diversifying your fat sources. Instead of slathering your bread with butter, try using avocado or olive oil. Use nuts and seeds as snacks instead of chips. Cooking at home with these healthier fats gives you control over what you consume. Replace the deep-fried foods with those that are baked or steamed and seasoned with healthy oils.

In an era where convenience foods dominate, it's easy to fall into the trap of processed oils and unhealthy fats. But, the effort to make these changes can have a profound impact on your health. That doesn't mean you need to eliminate all sources of saturated fat entirely, but rather, be mindful of how much and what kind you're consuming. For instance, high-quality grass-fed butter or coconut oil can be used sparingly as part of a diverse diet that includes plenty of monounsaturated and polyunsaturated fats.

As a health-conscious individual, parent, or even a healthcare professional, it's crucial to pass this knowledge on. Educate your children and community about the benefits of these fats. Involve them in cooking meals, choosing ingredients, and reading food labels. The collective effort to make healthier choices can lead to significant public health benefits over time.

For researchers and educators, the evolving science around dietary fats provides a rich area for continued study and public education. Ensuring that the latest findings are disseminated effectively can help counteract the myths and misconceptions that often surround discussions about dietary fats. It also adds a layer of credibility to dietary recommendations, which can sometimes feel overwhelming and contradictory to the general public.

In conclusion, understanding saturated, monounsaturated, and polyunsaturated fats is more than just an academic exercise. It is a practical tool for enhancing your diet and improving your health. By making informed choices and educating those around you, you can contribute to a broader shift toward healthier eating habits. Remember, the oils and fats you choose today can shape your health outcomes tomorrow.

Trans Fats and Hydrogenated Oils: The Hidden Dangers
Uncovering the veiled threats posed by trans fats and hydrogenated oils is crucial for anyone looking to adopt a healthier lifestyle. These ingredients lurk unnoticed in countless processed foods, from savory snacks to baked goods, and are more detrimental to your health than you may realize. To understand their risks, you have to know what they are, how they affect your body, and why steering clear of them can significantly improve your well-being.

Trans fats and hydrogenated oils are primarily found in processed and packaged foods. They were initially created to extend the shelf life of products and improve texture and flavor. However, these fats are far from beneficial. The hydrogenation process, introduced in the early 20th century, involves adding hydrogen molecules to vegetable oil to make it solid at room temperature, thus creating trans fats and partially hydrogenated oils (Mensink & Katan, 1990). Unfortunately, the very process designed to make foods last longer also turns them into health hazards.

One of the most alarming risks associated with trans fats is their impact on cardiovascular health. Multiple studies have shown that trans fats increase LDL cholesterol levels, the "bad" cholesterol, while simultaneously reducing HDL cholesterol, the "good" cholesterol. This double whammy significantly raises the risk of heart disease (Mozaffarian et al., 2006). For individuals already at risk—such as those with a family history of heart disease or existing cardiovascular issues—the consumption of trans fats can be particularly harmful. Trans fats also promote inflammation, which is a known factor in the development of numerous chronic diseases, including heart disease and diabetes (Mozaffarian et al., 2006).

The hidden danger of these fats is not just limited to cardiovascular health. They also play a significant role in metabolic disturbances and inflammation. Chronic inflammation caused by long-term consumption of trans fats can lead to conditions such as insulin resistance, paving the way for type 2 diabetes (Mozaffarian et al., 2006). Inflammation is the body's natural response to injury or infection, but when it becomes chronic due to poor dietary choices, it can wreak havoc on your system, contributing to a cascade of health issues.

If you're a parent, understanding the impact of trans fats and hydrogenated oils can help in making better choices for your children. Kids are often drawn to convenient snacks like cookies, crackers, and microwave popcorn, which are frequently loaded with these unhealthy fats. Regular consumption during childhood can set the foundation for poor health in adulthood, affecting everything from cardiovascular health to cognitive function (Smith, 2017).

Healthcare professionals frequently advise their patients to avoid foods containing trans fats and hydrogenated oils for a good reason. Long-term exposure to these fats doesn't just harm individual health; it also places a considerable burden on the healthcare system. Patients with chronic diseases often experience reduced quality of life and increased healthcare costs due to frequent medical visits, medications, and procedures (Mensink & Katan, 1990).

Switching to healthier fats doesn't have to be difficult. Reading food labels is the first step in avoiding trans fats and hydrogenated oils. Terms like "partially hydrogenated oil" in the ingredients list are red flags that should prompt you to put the product back on the shelf. Instead, opt for whole foods like avocados, nuts, and seeds for your fat intake. These natural sources provide essential nutrients that support your overall health.

Fitness enthusiasts might find that cutting out trans fats leads to improved performance and quicker recovery times. The inflammatory properties of trans fats can lead to sore muscles and extended recovery periods, hampering your progress and making workouts less enjoyable. Reducing or eliminating these fats from your diet can help you feel more energetic and less bogged down by inflammation.

But spotting these harmful fats isn't always straightforward. Food marketing can be misleading, and labels like "0 grams trans fat" can be deceptive. The FDA allows foods to be labeled as trans fat-free if they contain less than 0.5 grams of trans fat per serving. Consuming several servings can quickly add up, making it crucial to inspect ingredient lists carefully.

It's worth noting that restaurants and fast-food chains have historically been major culprits in using trans fats. Although many have moved toward healthier oils due to public pressure and legislative changes, menu items can still contain hidden trans fats. Being selective about where you dine and what you order can go a long way in reducing your intake of these damaging fats.

The ripple effects of these fats extend beyond individual health. The widespread use of trans fats in food products contributes to public health crises, affecting millions. Public health policies aimed at reducing trans fat intake, such as bans and labeling laws, have shown to be effective. For example, Denmark's trans fat ban led to a rapid and significant decrease in cardiovascular diseases among its population (Stender et al., 2006).

In summary, trans fats and hydrogenated oils represent hidden dangers that can have profound impacts on your health and well-being. They compromise cardiovascular health, promote systemic inflammation, and contribute to metabolic disorders. By educating yourself on how to avoid these harmful fats and making informed food choices, you can take a proactive stance in safeguarding your health and the health of your loved ones.

Chapter 4:
The Sugar Dilemma: Consumption and Health Risks

In today's fast-paced world, it's alarmingly easy to consume excessive amounts of sugar without even realizing it. The average diet is inundated with added sugars hiding in everything from breakfast cereals to savory sauces. This hidden sugar epidemic raises significant health concerns, linking overconsumption to a slew of chronic diseases like obesity, type 2 diabetes, and cardiovascular ailments (Johnson et al., 2009). As research continues to unravel the multifaceted risks associated with high sugar intake, it becomes clear that our dietary choices are directly impacting our overall well-being (Lustig, 2012). Balancing our sugar consumption is not just a matter of willpower but of making informed, intentional food choices that prioritize whole, unprocessed foods. By reducing sugar intake, we can foster better health outcomes, more stable energy levels, and a healthier relationship with food. Turning the tide on sugar consumption is not just a personal journey but a societal imperative, requiring education, mindfulness, and a proactive approach to one's diet (Te Morenga et al., 2013).

The Overconsumption Epidemic: How Much Sugar Is Too Much? We're living in an era where sugar has become a central character in our daily dramas. But just how much sugar is too much? This question isn't just about numbers and statistics; it's about the cumulative impact on our lives, our health, and the lives of our loved ones. What is it that makes excessive sugar such a pervasive issue despite overwhelming evidence of its health risks? To answer this question, we need to consider the broader cultural and economic factors at play, as well as the biological mechanisms that make sugar both desirable and detrimental.

First, let's address the scale of the problem. The average American consumes about 77 grams of sugar per day, equating to approximately 60 pounds per year (CDC, 2021). This is far above the recommended limits set by health organizations. The American Heart Association advises that men should not consume more than 36 grams (9 teaspoons) of added sugar per day, and women should limit their intake to 25 grams (6 teaspoons) (AHA, 2020). Why, then, is our consumption so staggeringly high?

One reason lies in the insidious presence of sugar in nearly every processed food we consume. From the obvious culprits like candies and sodas to the less obvious such as bread, sauces, and even "healthy" snacks like granola bars, sugar sneaks into our diets in multiple ways. Food companies often use sugar not only to enhance flavor but also as a preservative and texturizer, making it an almost indispensable ingredient in processed foods (Lustig, 2012).

But it's not just about external factors; there's a biological element that influences our sugar consumption, too. Sugar impacts our brain in much the same way as addictive substances, releasing dopamine and creating a sense of pleasure and reward. This profound impact on the brain's reward system can make cutting back on sugar incredibly challenging (DiNicolantonio et al., 2018).

The body's metabolic response to sugar overconsumption is equally concerning. High sugar intake leads to spikes in blood glucose levels, which in turn prompts the release of insulin. Over time, this can cause insulin resistance, a precursor to type 2 diabetes (Stanhope, 2016). Moreover, excessive sugar has been linked to obesity, cardiovascular diseases, and a slew of other metabolic syndromes (Hu, 2013).

So, how do we calibrate our sugar intake to align with these health guidelines? Awareness is the first step. Reading food labels carefully helps in making informed decisions. Many labels now list added sugars separately, making it easier to track and reduce intake. Cooking at home using whole ingredients can also give better control over the amount of sugar in meals.

This challenge extends to parents striving to set a healthy example for their children. Kids are particularly vulnerable to the adverse effects of sugar because their taste preferences and eating habits are formed early on. High sugar consumption in childhood has been linked to increased risks of obesity, type 2 diabetes, and even cognitive impairments later in life (Vos et al., 2017). Creating a balanced diet for children that limits added sugars can help mitigate these risks.

For those with specific health conditions like diabetes or cardiovascular diseases, moderating sugar intake is not just advisable; it's essential. Cutting down on sugar can be a life-saving adjustment. It's crucial to replace empty calories from sugar with nutrient-rich alternatives like fruits, vegetables, and whole grains. These offer not just sustenance but also essential vitamins, minerals, and fibers that are often missing in high-sugar diets (Johnson et al., 2009).

Moreover, the role of healthcare professionals and educators cannot be understated in this battle. They can guide individuals through the maze of food choices and offer personalized advice based on one's health status and lifestyle. Public health campaigns and educational programs aimed at reducing sugar consumption have shown promising results, indicating that a collective effort can indeed make a significant impact (WHO, 2015).

How much sugar is too much? The answer isn't a simple number but a more intricate balancing act involving awareness, education, and intentional choices. By understanding the profound effects of sugar and taking actionable steps to limit it, we move closer to a healthier, more vibrant life. As we navigate our dietary choices, let's keep this in mind: every small cutback on sugar is a giant leap toward improved health and well-being for us and our families.

If you're inspired by what you've read and find the information valuable, your online review would mean the world to us. Your feedback helps in reaching more people who could benefit from understanding and managing their sugar intake. Together, we can create a ripple effect, encouraging healthier choices and fostering a community committed to better health.

Sweet Diseases: Linking Sugar to Health Conditions encompasses a critical examination of how excessive sugar consumption impacts our health. One of the major concerns today is the staggering rise in chronic diseases directly correlated with modern dietary habits, particularly high sugar intake. From obesity to type 2 diabetes, cardiovascular diseases to certain types of cancer, the evidence supporting the deleterious health effects of sugar is both robust and compelling (Malik et al., 2010). This section serves as a bridge in our narrative, vividly illustrating the link between sugar and various health conditions, which are of paramount concern to not just adults but children and adolescents alike.

Let's start with obesity. There's no denying the epidemic proportions of obesity worldwide, and sugar, especially the hidden high-fructose corn syrup in many processed foods, plays a starring role. Unlike glucose, which our bodies can utilize effectively, fructose is metabolized in the liver where it can lead to increased fat production (Stanhope, 2012). Obesity is more than just an aesthetic issue; it's a gateway condition that predisposes individuals to a slate of other serious health complications, including heart disease, stroke, and type 2 diabetes.

The connection between sugar and type 2 diabetes is another critical area where awareness is key. Consistent overconsumption of sugar can cause insulin resistance, a hallmark of type 2 diabetes. Insulin resistance means that your cells become less responsive to insulin, compelling your pancreas to produce more to manage blood glucose levels. Over time, this relentless demand on the pancreas can lead to its dysfunction, resulting in chronically high blood sugar levels and diabetes (Hu, 2011). By reducing sugar intake, you can significantly decrease your risk of developing this debilitating condition.

Cardiovascular health is also under siege from excessive sugar consumption. High sugar intake has been linked to increased levels of triglycerides and LDL cholesterol, both markers of cardiovascular disease (Johnson et al., 2009). Moreover, sugar can raise blood pressure and promote inflammation, compounding the risk of heart ailments. A heart-healthy diet isn't just about cutting out fats; it's also about recognizing and eliminating the sugars that we unwittingly consume in significant quantities every day.

Cancer is yet another area where sugar's impact demands attention. Some research suggests that high insulin levels associated with sugar intake may promote the growth of certain cancer cells. Insulin is a growth factor, and in high quantities, it can potentially encourage the proliferation of cancer cells (Gatenby & Gillies, 2004). While more research is needed to conclusively establish this link, the preliminary evidence already justifies caution and moderation in sugar consumption.

Beyond the diseases traditionally associated with sugar, there's a growing body of evidence linking sugar to non-alcoholic fatty liver disease (NAFLD). Fructose, in particular, is implicated in the development of NAFLD because it's metabolized almost exclusively in the liver, where it can be converted to fat (Sanyal, 2019). Overconsumption can burden the liver, leading to fat accumulation and ultimately liver inflammation and damage.

Mental health also hasn't escaped the shadow of sugar. Emerging research suggests that high sugar intake can exacerbate symptoms of anxiety and depression. The inflammation and oxidative stress prompted by sugar can affect brain function, potentially leading to mood disorders (Westover & Marangell, 2002). Thus, reducing sugar isn't just about physical health but mental well-being too.

For parents and educators, these revelations are essential when considering the diet of children and teenagers. Recent studies highlight a disturbing increase in childhood obesity and type 2 diabetes, conditions once rare in young populations (Han et al., 2010). The health patterns established during childhood often persist into adulthood, underscoring the importance of instilling healthier eating habits early on. By addressing the sugar content in children's diets, we can mitigate future health risks and cultivate a generation better equipped to make informed dietary choices.

As we consider these applications to different audiences—whether healthcare professionals advising patients, fitness enthusiasts optimizing performance, or parents nurturing healthy kids—the unifying theme is clear: excessive sugar has far-reaching negative health implications. Educating oneself about these risks and making informed dietary adjustments can substantially improve overall well-being.

In our modern food landscape dense with added sugars, it's imperative to stay vigilant. Educational initiatives aimed at deciphering food labels and recognizing hidden sugars can empower consumers to make healthier choices. The responsibility of educating the public falls on healthcare professionals, educators, and even authors committed to disseminating clear, evidence-based information.

As you move through the chapters and sections of this book, let the insights gained here lay a firm foundation upon which you build a healthier dietary regime. The next time you reach for a sugary snack, remember the hidden costs that such indulgences may exact on your health. Armed with knowledge and motivation, you've taken the first step toward a sugar-moderated lifestyle. Each small step counts towards a significant impact on your overall health.

To ensure that others also benefit from this critical information, we encourage you to share your thoughts and experiences. The next section titled **Online Review Request for This Book** provides an opportunity for you to contribute your voice to the ongoing dialogue about sugar and its impact on health. Your feedback can help spread awareness and foster a community committed to making healthier, informed choices.

Chapter 5:
Oily Issues: How Processed Fats Affect Our Bodies

Processed fats, often lurking in everyday foods, are more than just a dietary inconvenience—they're a significant health threat. When we consume these fats, such as those found in hydrogenated oils and margarine, our bodies respond with inflammation, a key contributor to chronic diseases like diabetes, obesity, and arthritis (Mozaffarian et al., 2006). Unlike natural, unprocessed fats, processed fats disrupt our metabolic systems, leading to increased risk of cardiovascular diseases (Mensink et al., 2003). This isn't just about weight—it's about foundational health issues that impact every part of our lives. Understanding the science behind these fats empowers us to make better choices, replacing harmful oils with healthier alternatives, thus fostering better long-term health and vitality (Jacobson & Willett, 2009).

The Inflammatory Response: Connecting Oils to Chronic Diseases oil consumption isn't just about extra calories or heart disease risk. The type of oil you eat can profoundly influence inflammation in your body—a root cause of many chronic diseases like diabetes, arthritis, and even Alzheimer's. But how do processed fats make this happen? Understanding this connection can empower you to make healthier choices and improve your long-term well-being significantly.

Inflammation is part of your body's natural healing process, but when it becomes chronic, it wreaks havoc on tissues and organs.

Chronic inflammation has been linked to numerous diseases, including cardiovascular disease, type 2 diabetes, and certain cancers (Hotamisligil, 2006). So how do processed oils contribute to this type of harmful, persistent inflammation? One significant factor is the imbalance of omega-6 to omega-3 fatty acids in the typical Western diet.

Omega-6 fatty acids are crucial for human health, but the modern diet often contains them in excessive amounts due to the prevalent use of vegetable oils like soybean, corn, and sunflower oil (Simopoulos, 2002). Unlike the balanced ratio of omega-3 and omega-6 found in traditional diets, modern diets can have ratios skewed as high as 20:1 in favor of omega-6s. This imbalance promotes the production of pro-inflammatory cytokines, which can aggravate chronic inflammation (Calder, 2008).

Beyond the omega imbalance, another concerning aspect is how these oils are processed. Many vegetable oils undergo high heat, chemical treatments, and deodorization, altering their structure. This processing often creates trans fats, harmful compounds linked to elevated inflammation markers like C-reactive protein (CRP) (Mozaffarian et al., 2006). It's not just the trans fats; other byproducts formed during high-heat processing, such as oxidized lipids, are also problematic. These oxidized compounds are extremely inflammatory and can contribute to insulin resistance, a precursor to type 2 diabetes (Devaraj et al., 2008).

It's critical to look at the bigger picture. Yes, skipping processed oils can help reduce inflammation, but incorporating anti-inflammatory foods is essential too. For instance, cold-water fish, flaxseeds, and walnuts can help balance your omega-6 and omega-3 ratio. These foods are rich in alpha-linolenic acid (ALA), an omega-3 fatty acid that has been shown to reduce markers of inflammation

(Gemini et al., 2015). Even switching to extra virgin olive oil, rich in anti-inflammatory polyphenols, can make a significant difference.

When we discuss chronic inflammation, it's essential to understand it's not just an abstract concept confined to scientific journals. The practical implications are profound. Chronic inflammation silently damages tissues over time, setting the stage for diseases that decrease the quality of life. For instance, consider type 2 diabetes. The relationship between inflammation and insulin resistance is well-documented. As inflammation increases, insulin's ability to regulate blood sugar decreases, paving the way for diabetes (Shoelson et al., 2006).

The heart is another organ that bears the brunt of a high-inflammatory diet. Pro-inflammatory cytokines can contribute to the buildup of arterial plaque, leading to atherosclerosis—a significant risk factor for heart attacks and strokes (Libby, 2002). This isn't just about numbers and statistics; it's about real-world impacts on you and the people you love. Think about the devastating effects of a heart attack or stroke, not just on the individual but also on their families.

Switching gears, let's touch upon how inflammation impacts neurological health. Emerging studies suggest that neuroinflammation might play a crucial role in Alzheimer's disease. A diet high in pro-inflammatory fats can exacerbate this inflammation, accelerating cognitive decline (Kanoski & Davidson, 2011). The brain is highly susceptible to oxidative stress and inflammation, so the food choices you make today could significantly impact your cognitive health down the line.

So, what can you do to mitigate these risks? First, re-evaluate the oils you use in your kitchen. Opt for oils with a better profile, like extra virgin olive oil or avocado oil. Use them within their smoke points to avoid the formation of harmful compounds. When possible, aim to cook at lower temperatures to preserve the beneficial properties of these oils. Also, include more whole foods like leafy greens, nuts, seeds, and fatty fish in your diet to naturally combat inflammation.

We can't ignore the role of labeling and food manufacturing practices in all this. Often, processed foods contain hidden oils that contribute to your daily intake of omega-6 fatty acids without you even realizing it. Learning to read labels carefully and making informed choices can help you sidestep these hidden pitfalls. Seek out products that are minimally processed and free of hydrogenated or partially hydrogenated oils.

Beyond individual changes, advocating for better food policies and supporting brands that prioritize health over profit can create broader systemic changes. As more consumers demand healthier oils and fewer inflammatories in processed foods, companies will have to adapt to maintain their market share.

In conclusion, understanding the inflammatory response and its connection to oils is more than just scientific curiosity—it's a pivotal step in reclaiming your health. Small but consistent changes in your diet can lead to remarkable improvements over time. By focusing on reducing harmful oils and incorporating more anti-inflammatory foods, you can pave the way for a healthier, longer life. It's about taking control, making informed choices, and inspiring others to do the same.

Remember, every positive change you make sends ripples through your life and the lives of those around you. We hope you find this information enlightening and empowering, and if you do, we'd appreciate it if you could take a moment to leave an **Online Review for This Book**. Your feedback helps us reach a broader audience and fosters a community focused on better health and well-being.

Heart of the Matter: Processed Oils and Cardiovascular Health are significant areas of concern in modern dietary practices.

The impact of processed oils on cardiovascular health is both profound and often underestimated. By exploring the intricate relationship between these oils and heart health, we can better understand their role and mitigate potential risks.

Processed oils, such as hydrogenated oils and those high in trans fats, have been shown to contribute significantly to cardiovascular diseases (CVD). Studies consistently demonstrate that these oils can increase LDL (low-density lipoprotein) cholesterol levels while decreasing HDL (high-density lipoprotein) cholesterol levels, a combination that heightens the risk of heart disease (Mensink & Katan, 1990). The mechanism here is that trans fats alter the lipid profile, leading to arterial plaque buildup, which can obstruct blood flow and elevate blood pressure, ultimately escalating the risk of heart attacks and strokes.

Remarkably, the body of evidence is not just limited to cholesterol modulation. Processed oils also induce an inflammatory response, which is another critical pathway leading to cardiovascular health degradation (Mozaffarian et al., 2006). Inflammation within the blood vessels can cause damage that predisposes these vessels to atherosclerosis—the buildup of fats, cholesterol, and other substances in and on the artery walls. This leads to restricted blood flow, increasing the risk of CVD.

Incorporating highly processed oils into our diets isn't just about poor cholesterol levels or inflammation. These oils are often found in processed foods that also contain high amounts of sugar and salt, forming a triple threat to cardiovascular health. The synergy of high processed oil, sugar, and salt intake can exacerbate hypertension and other metabolic syndromes, furthering the risk of developing heart conditions (Micha & Mozaffarian, 2010).

Interestingly, lifestyle changes focused on reducing processed oil intake can have immediate and significant impacts on overall heart health. Numerous intervention studies have underscored that replacing trans fats with healthier fats, such as those found in olive oil or avocados, can markedly improve cardiovascular outcomes (Katan et al., 1995). Substituting these harmful fats with omega-3 and omega-6 fatty acids—which offer protective benefits for the heart—can bring about an increase in HDL cholesterol while lowering LDL cholesterol and triglycerides, further curbing inflammation and stabilizing heart rhythm.

Translating these scientific insights into practical dietary changes is crucial. For those striving to improve their cardiovascular health, it's essential to be aware of the types of oils in their diet. Favor oils such as olive oil, coconut oil in moderation, and oils rich in omega-3 fatty acids. Avoid items hydrogenated or partially hydrogenated oils, commonly listed in ingredient labels, to mitigate the risks of cardiovascular ailments.

Applying this knowledge can indeed transform lives. It's not just about cutting out certain oils but replacing them with better alternatives, which can help break the cycle of poor heart health caused by processed oils. For instance, if you're accustomed to using vegetable oil in your salad dressing, consider switching to extra virgin olive oil. Similarly, swap out margarine for real butter or a plant-based alternative that doesn't contain hydrogenated oils. These small but meaningful adjustments can drastically improve cardiovascular health in the long run (Hu et al., 2001).

Moreover, public health initiatives aimed at reducing trans fat consumption have led to positive outcomes worldwide. Countries that have restricted or banned the use of hydrogenated oils have seen a decline in cardiovascular disease rates. This demonstrates that policy changes—and individual actions—can create a ripple effect, fostering healthier communities (Downs et al., 2013).

Yet, the battle against processed oils is far from won. Food manufacturers continue to exploit consumer ignorance by substituting one harmful oil with another or by not being transparent about their use of such oils. This makes it incumbent on us, as informed consumers, to diligently read labels and stay abreast of the ever-evolving list of ingredients used in our foods. Empowering ourselves with knowledge remains a vital step toward protecting our cardiovascular health.

Through conscious dietary choices geared toward reducing or eliminating processed oils, you can pave the way for improved heart health, greater energy levels, and a higher quality of life. Make it a collective effort—encourage friends and family to be mindful of their oil intake. Together, small changes can culminate in remarkable strides against cardiovascular diseases.

As we wind down the discussion on the detrimental effects of processed oils on cardiovascular health, remember how knowledge can become a powerful tool. The journey toward improved heart health can be an enriching experience, empowering you to make better choices for yourself and your loved ones. Share this wisdom, and let's foster a heart-healthy world, one oil choice at a time.

Chapter 6:
Sugar and Kids: Setting Up for a Healthy Future

In today's world, children are constantly bombarded with sugary temptations, posing a significant challenge for parents trying to foster healthy eating habits. Excessive sugar intake can have detrimental effects on a child's development, impacting cognitive function, mood, and long-term metabolic health (Goran et al., 2013). Setting children up for a healthy future involves implementing practical strategies to reduce sugar consumption without sacrificing joy and flavor. This may include educating kids about the health impacts of sugar, encouraging the consumption of whole foods, and fostering an environment where nutritious choices are both accessible and appealing. By teaching children to appreciate the natural sweetness in fruits and understanding the adverse effects of sugar-laden snacks, parents can nurture lifelong habits that protect against obesity, diabetes, and other metabolic disorders (Johnson et al., 2007). This chapter delves into evidence-based approaches to minimize sugar in children's diets, emphasizing the importance of making these changes a family affair to ensure consistency and support.

The Impact of Sweet Foods on Child Development is a crucial aspect of ensuring our children's long-term health and well-being. As parents and caregivers, it's essential to understand how sugary foods influence various aspects of a child's growth. High-sugar diets can have negative implications on physical health, cognitive development, and emotional well-being. Too often, the appeal of sweetness masks the potential detrimental effects sugar has on the developing bodies and minds of our children.

Our lives are inundated with convenience foods loaded with added sugars. Items like breakfast cereals, fruit snacks, beverages, and even seemingly healthy choices like yogurt can harbor surprising amounts of sugar. The implications of regular consumption of these sugary foods go well beyond occasional indulgence. Excessive sugar intake in children has been linked to an increased risk of developing obesity, diabetes, and dental cavities (Moynihan & Kelly, 2014).

Physically, children consuming high amounts of sugar can experience rapid weight gain. Obesity rates in children have skyrocketed, and sugary diets play a significant role. Children with a high-sugar diet tend to have more body fat, leading to a higher body mass index (BMI). This excessive weight can lead to metabolic disorders such as type 2 diabetes—a condition that was once almost unheard of in children but is now increasingly diagnosed (Hu et al., 2019).

Additionally, sugar can compromise bone density. Studies suggest that children consuming diets rich in sugary beverages have lower bone density, which could affect their overall growth. It's believed that high sugar intake might interfere with the absorption of critical nutrients like calcium and magnesium, both of which are vital for bone health (Libuda ct al., 2008).

Cognitive development also suffers. Diets high in sugar have been associated with impeded learning abilities and memory issues in children. Research has shown that high sugar intake can lead to reduced cognitive functioning and a decline in attention span. The mechanisms behind this are still being studied, but evidence suggests that sugar may negatively impact synaptic plasticity and neurogenesis—the processes crucial for learning and memory formation (Noble & Kanoski, 2016).

In terms of emotional well-being, sugar can play a tricky role. While a sugar rush might result in temporary hyperactivity, it's often followed by a "crash," manifesting as mood swings or irritability. Over time, high sugar consumption can contribute to behavioral issues. Some studies have linked high sugar intake to an increased risk of developing attention deficit hyperactivity disorder (ADHD) and increased anxiety levels. It's essential to consider how sugar impacts a child's mood and behavior, as these factors dramatically influence their daily lives and interactions (Millichap & Yee, 2012).

A critical concern is the development of taste preferences. Children exposed to high levels of sugar early on may develop a strong preference for sugary foods, making it difficult for them to enjoy healthier options later. This palate conditioning can create long-term eating habits that favor sugary foods over nutrient-dense options like fruits, vegetables, and whole grains. Ensuring a balance in early childhood diets can set the stage for healthier food preferences throughout life.

Another aspect worth discussing is the hidden sugar found in supposed "healthy" foods. Items marketed toward children, often adorned with vibrant colors and cartoon characters, can contain shocking amounts of added sugars. Parents must become adept at reading nutritional labels to identify these hidden sugars, ensuring they make informed decisions about their children's nutritional intake. Limiting these harmful additives can contribute significantly to better overall health outcomes (Lustig, 2012).

Educators and healthcare professionals have a pivotal role in addressing this epidemic. They must emphasize the importance of a balanced diet rich in whole foods and low in added sugars. Schools can incorporate nutrition education into their curriculums, teaching children the value of healthy eating habits from a young age. Independent and sponsored research also brings light to the profound effects of sugar on child development, giving parents and caregivers actionable insights (Reilly & Kelly, 2011).

Building a foundation of healthy eating habits is a community effort involving schools, healthcare providers, and families working together. Encouraging children to participate in meal planning and preparation can make them more invested in their dietary choices. Educating children about the benefits of various food groups and the detriments of excessive sugar can empower them to make healthier decisions independently.

The journey to reducing sugar in children's diets is challenging but rewarding. Each small step, whether it's swapping a sugary snack for a piece of fruit or educating kids about the dangers of excessive sugar, contributes to a healthier future. Together, we can combat the impact of sugary foods on child development and pave the way for healthier generations to come.

As we conclude this section, remember to apply this information holistically and share your experiences and insights. Your feedback is invaluable not just to us, but to other readers who can learn from your journey. Be sure to leave a review of this book in the "Online Review Request for This Book" section to help spread the message and further our shared goal of enhancing child health.

Creating Sweet Change: Reducing Sugar in Kid's Diets is vital to ensuring a healthy future for our children. In today's fast-paced world, filled with convenient yet sugar-laden foods, parents face a significant challenge: how to reduce sugar in their kids' diets without causing stress or rebellion. The key lies in gradual, thoughtful changes that empower both parents and children to make healthier choices together.

First and foremost, it's essential to recognize the profound effects of excessive sugar consumption on children's health. Numerous studies have shown a strong correlation between high sugar intake and adverse health outcomes like obesity, type 2 diabetes, and dental problems (Lustig, 2012). Additionally, sugar has been linked to behavioral issues and poor academic performance, making it all the more crucial for parents to take actionable steps (Wolraich et al., 1994).

One practical approach to reducing sugar intake is to start by limiting sugary beverages, such as sodas, fruit juices, and energy drinks. These account for a significant portion of added sugars in the average child's diet. Encouraging children to drink water, milk, or unsweetened herbal teas can drastically reduce their daily sugar consumption. Substituting flavored water with slices of fruits or herbs, like mint, can make the transition more appealing.

When it comes to meals and snacks, aim to increase the proportion of whole foods. Whole fruits, for example, are far better options than fruit snacks or sugary desserts. They provide essential nutrients and fiber, which help regulate blood sugar levels, reducing the likelihood of sugar spikes that can lead to crashes and mood swings. By presenting fruits in fun and creative ways—such as fruit kebabs or mixed fruit salads—you can make them more enticing to young palates.

Revising family recipes is another excellent strategy for cutting down sugar intake. Substitute refined sugars with natural sweeteners like honey, maple syrup, or mashed fruits such as bananas and applesauce. While still sweet, these substitutes offer added nutritional benefits and a lower glycemic index compared to processed sugars. For instance, swapping half the sugar in a muffin recipe with applesauce can reduce the overall sugar content while maintaining sweetness and moisture.

Educational engagement is crucial for long-term success. Teaching kids about the consequences of high sugar consumption empowers them to make informed decisions. One effective method is involving them in food preparation. When kids help cook, they become more aware of the ingredients and can see firsthand the amount of sugar that goes into recipes. This hands-on experience can foster healthier eating habits and a greater appreciation for nutritious foods.

Schools also play an essential role in shaping children's dietary habits. Advocating for healthier school lunch programs and snack options can reinforce the steps taken at home. Collaborating with teachers and school administrators to create a supportive environment ensures consistent messaging about the importance of reducing sugar intake.

Finally, awareness of deceptive marketing strategies is critical. Many products labeled as "low-fat" or "healthy" often compensate with added sugars to enhance flavor (Te Morenga, Mallard, & Mann, 2013). Learning to read and understand food labels can help parents make more informed choices. Look for terms like "high fructose corn syrup," "sucrose," "glucose," and "maltose" as indicators of added sugars in products.

Creating sweet change in kids' diets is not about deprivation but about making smarter choices that lead to lasting health benefits. By gradually reducing sugar intake and fostering an environment that values whole foods, we can guide our children toward a healthier, more balanced lifestyle. This collective effort, supported by both parents and educators, ensures that we set the best possible foundation for our children's future health and well-being.

Ultimately, it's a journey that requires patience, persistence, and a willingness to adapt. But the rewards—a generation of healthier, more informed children—are well worth the effort.

Chapter 7:
Fat Facts: The Role of Oils
in Child Nutrition

As we delve into the vital role of oils in child nutrition, it's essential to recognize that fats aren't the villains they're often made out to be. They're indispensable for the physical and cognitive development of growing bodies. The right types of fats—namely those derived from whole, unprocessed oils like extra virgin olive oil, avocado oil, and even certain animal fats—provide crucial nutrients that support cell membranes, hormone production, and brain health (DeBose et al., 2020). However, the key lies in discerning the beneficial fats from the harmful ones. Introducing children to healthy oils early in life sets a foundation for long-term well-being. Notably, omega-3 and omega-6 fatty acids play a crucial role in brain development and function, underscoring the need for strategic dietary choices (Simopoulos, 2002). Ultimately, educating parents and caregivers about the importance of selecting high-quality oils can lead to healthier eating habits that benefit children throughout their lives.

The Need for Fat in Growing Bodies is an incredibly essential topic that often gets overshadowed by the stereotypical fear of fat in our diets. While adults might be worried about the implications of high-fat intake, children's nutritional needs tell a different story. Let's explore why fat is not just beneficial but critical for growing bodies.

right fats can greatly influence brain development in children. During the early years of life, the brain grows at an unprecedented rate, and healthy fats are a necessity for this development. Essential fatty acids, such as omega-3s, are significant in supporting the structure and functioning of brain cell membranes (Rettner, 2014). These fats not only foster cognitive development but also play a role in improving attention and behavior. It's no coincidence that children who consume diets rich in healthy fats tend to perform better cognitively and emotionally. Therefore, ensuring kids have access to high-quality oils rich in omega-3s could very well pave the way for a brighter, more focused future.

Moreover, fat serves as a concentrated source of energy, crucial for the hyperactive lifestyles children lead. Kids are constantly moving—from playgrounds to sports fields, they burn an enormous amount of energy. Fats offer twice the energy per gram as carbohydrates or proteins, ensuring they have enough fuel to sustain their activity levels. Imagine a child, akin to a high-performance car. Would you fuel a race car with low-quality gasoline? No. The same logic applies to children; they need high-quality fats for optimal performance and growth.

Also, fats are integral for the absorption of essential fat-soluble vitamins like vitamins A, D, E, and K. These vitamins play multifaceted roles in immune function, bone health, and cellular protection. For instance, Vitamin A is vital for vision, while Vitamin D is crucial for strong bones and immune health. Without adequate fat in their diet, children wouldn't be able to absorb these vitamins efficiently, potentially leading to deficiencies and related health issues. This underscores the importance of incorporating healthy fats into their daily regimen.

A common concern among parents is calories and weight management. It's essential to understand that not all fats lead to weight gain. Diets high in trans fats and unhealthy processed fats can indeed contribute to obesity, but healthy fats from sources like avocados, nuts, seeds, and olive oil do not have the same effect. In fact, these healthier fats can satiate hunger more effectively than their processed counterparts, helping kids avoid constant snacking and leading to more balanced eating habits (Dashti et al., 2017).

Another critical aspect worth noting is the role of fats in hormonal development. Fats are fundamental in the formation of hormones, which are crucial for growth and puberty. Cholesterol, often misunderstood and demonized, is actually a building block for hormones like estrogen and testosterone. This is why kids, especially those in their adolescent years, need an ample supply of healthy fats to go through these vital developmental stages smoothly.

We also cannot ignore the cultural aspect. In many traditional diets around the world, fats have been a staple, especially in nutrition for children. Take the Mediterranean diet, renowned for its health benefits, which places a high emphasis on healthy fats from fish, olive oil, and nuts. These dietary patterns often come with lower rates of chronic diseases and healthier weights among children, making a compelling case for the inclusion of good fats in our diets (Willett et al., 1995).

Yet, navigating the world of fats can be confusing. Parents are bombarded with conflicting information and it's easy to fall into the trap of low-fat diets, believing they're doing their children a favor. However, armed with the right information, you can make choices that will benefit your children both in their immediate growth and long-term health. The key lies in opting for healthy fats and steering clear of trans fats and overly processed oils.

Sources that are excellent for children include fatty fish like salmon, known for its high omega-3 content; seeds and nuts, which offer a good mix of healthy fatty acids; avocados, filled with monounsaturated fats; and oils like olive and flaxseed oil. These choices ensure that kids get their requisite fat intake without the associated risks that come with unhealthy alternatives.

As we move to the overarching mission of this book, it's evident that education is vital. We aim to shift the narrative around fats and impart that, particularly for children, fats are friends, not foes. By making informed decisions, we can ensure that our children grow up strong, healthy, and ready to tackle whatever the future holds.

As you delve deeper into subsequent sections, like "Choosing the Right Oils for Healthy Development," we'll provide practical tips and deeper insights on integrating these concepts into everyday life. We'll show you how to shop smart, cook healthily, and balance dietary needs without sacrificing flavor. After all, a healthy diet is a cornerstone of a happy, vibrant life.

Ensuring we grasp "The Need for Fat in Growing Bodies" not only empowers parents to make better dietary choices but also supports enduring well-being. With a keen understanding of the roles fats play, you will be better equipped to foster environments where healthy growth is paramount.

Choosing the Right Oils for Healthy Development is pivotal to ensure that our children grow up with robust bodies and vibrant minds. Oils and fats are essential components of a child's diet, contributing significantly to growth and development. But not all oils are created equal. Choosing the right types of oils can make all the difference in fostering a healthy future for our children.

First and foremost, it's crucial to understand that healthy fats are necessary for brain development. The brain is made up mostly of fat, particularly omega-3 and omega-6 fatty acids, which play a fundamental role in cognitive functions and overall brain health (Innis, 2007). Therefore, incorporating oils rich in these fatty acids is paramount. Sources such as flaxseed oil, fish oil, and walnut oil are excellent providers of omega-3s, while oils like sunflower and safflower oil offer omega-6s.

Incorporating monounsaturated fats is another important aspect. Oils such as olive oil and avocado oil are rich in monounsaturated fats, which help promote heart health by reducing bad cholesterol levels. Research has consistently shown that diets high in monounsaturated fats can reduce the risk of cardiovascular diseases (Mensink, 2001). These oils also provide Vitamin E, a potent antioxidant that protects cells from damage and supports immune function. Including these oils in your child's diet can be as simple as using them in salad dressings or for light sautéing of vegetables.

Moreover, let's discuss the polyunsaturated fats, which include essential fatty acids that our bodies can't produce on their own. Essential fatty acids are critical for cell membrane production and hormone regulation. Fish oil is an exceptional source of these fats, particularly DHA and EPA, which are linked to improved cognitive function and reduced inflammation. For children who might be picky eaters, flavored fish oil supplements can be a workaround.

While these are the beneficial fats, it's equally important to avoid certain harmful oils. Trans fats, largely found in hydrogenated oils, are particularly damaging. They not only raise bad cholesterol levels but also lower good cholesterol, leading to increased risks of heart disease, diabetes, and other chronic conditions (Mozaffarian et al., 2006). These are often hidden in processed foods, so steering clear of items like margarine, baked goods, and fried foods can significantly benefit your child's health. Always check labels for partially hydrogenated oils and aim to eliminate them from your family's diet.

Aside from the types of fats, the quality of the oils we use is essential. Opt for cold-pressed, extra virgin, and unrefined oils whenever possible, as these retain more of the beneficial nutrients compared to their refined counterparts. Cooking at lower temperatures helps preserve these nutrients. For high-heat cooking, it's better to use oils with higher smoke points like avocado oil or ghee, which maintain their integrity and nutritional value even when heated.

Including a variety of oils can also ensure that children get a more balanced intake of fatty acids. Blending different oils in cooking can introduce unique flavors and a broader array of nutrients. A byproduct of this variety is that it keeps meals interesting, making it easier to maintain these healthier choices.

Adjusting to healthier oils doesn't mean compromising on taste or creativity in the kitchen. Simple swaps like replacing butter with olive oil in baking or using coconut oil for a subtle tropical flavor can deliver health benefits without sacrificing flavor. Engaging children in the process of cooking and educating them about the benefits of these oils can cultivate lifelong healthy eating habits.

To aid in making these choices, it's beneficial to educate ourselves continually. This includes reading up-to-date research, consulting with healthcare professionals, and staying aware of new information. Resources such as the American Heart Association provide guidelines and recommendations that are based on the latest scientific research.

Ultimately, creating a diet rich in healthy oils can set the foundation for a lifetime of well-being for our children. By consciously making better choices, we empower not just our kids but also ourselves, steering our families toward healthier, happier lives.

Chapter 8:
Reading Between the Labels:
Identifying Hidden Sugars and Fats

Understanding the intricacies of food labels is crucial in today's world, where added sugars and unhealthy fats can be disguised under a plethora of names. Many consumers are unaware that ingredients like "evaporated cane juice" or "agave nectar" are just alternate names for sugar, while terms like "partially hydrogenated oils" indicate the presence of trans fats. Food manufacturers often exploit these aliases to market their products as healthier than they truly are, leading to unintentional consumption of harmful substances (Lustig, 2012; Mozaffarian et al., 2010). By becoming adept at decoding labels, individuals can make more informed choices, avoiding the health pitfalls associated with these hidden additives ("Mozaffarian et al., 2010). This chapter will empower readers with the knowledge to navigate food labels confidently, fostering better dietary habits that contribute to overall well-being.

Deciphering Food Labels: A Guide to Informed Choices might seem daunting, with the endless jargon and unpronounceable ingredients. But this skill is the gateway to making healthier choices for yourself and your family. Food labels are not just legal necessities; they are treasure troves of information waiting to be unlocked. By understanding these labels, you make informed decisions that align with your health goals and well-being.

Understanding food labels begins with recognizing the various types of sugars and fats hiding in your food. These ingredients are often cloaked under various names that can be confusing for the average consumer. For instance, sugars can appear as fructose, glucose, sucrose, or even corn syrup. Fats, on the other hand, can be shown as hydrogenated oils, partially hydrogenated oils, or trans fats. Knowing these aliases helps you avoid unwanted additions to your diet that might derail your health journey (Lustig, 2013; Willett et al., 2019).

One essential aspect of deciphering food labels is understanding the serving size. Manufacturers often use smaller serving sizes to make the nutritional content appear more favorable. By comparing the serving size to the portion you actually consume, you get a more accurate picture of how much sugar and fat you're ingesting. This practice is particularly crucial when looking at snacks and packaged foods where the serving sizes are often misleadingly small (Nestle, 2013).

Nutrition Facts Panel is where most of your attention should be focused. This section provides a detailed breakdown of the calories, macronutrients, and micronutrients in the food item. Pay special attention to the amount of added sugars and the types of fats listed. Government guidelines recommend limiting added sugars to less than 10% of your total daily calories. This equates to roughly 50 grams of sugar on a 2,000-calorie diet (American Heart Association, 2023).

The ingredient list is another crucial part of the food label. Ingredients are listed in descending order by weight. The sooner an ingredient appears on the list, the more of that ingredient is present in the product. If sugars or unhealthy oils dominate the top of the ingredient list, it's a red flag that the product might not be the healthiest choice for you. Remember, words like "evaporated cane juice," "agave nectar," and "brown rice syrup" are just euphemisms for sugar (Teicholz, 2014).

Beware of Marketing Gimmicks on food packages. Terms like "all-natural," "low-fat," or "fat-free" can be misleading. These labels can create a halo effect, making you believe the product is healthier than it is. For example, "low-fat" products often contain added sugars to compensate for the loss of flavor that comes with reduced fat content. Similarly, "all-natural" doesn't necessarily mean the product is healthy; it just means that the ingredients are derived from natural sources. Always cross-check these claims with the Nutrition Facts Panel and the ingredient list to get the full story (Ludwig & Nestle, 2008).

For those with specific health conditions, such as diabetes or cardiovascular issues, reading food labels becomes even more critical. Not all fats are created equal, and some, like trans fats, can exacerbate health problems. Trans fats increase bad LDL cholesterol and decrease good HDL cholesterol, contributing to heart disease. They are often found in processed foods, so zeroing in on any mention of "hydrogenated" or "partially hydrogenated" oils in the ingredient list is essential for making heart-healthy choices (Fung & Hu, 2003).

Understanding Percent Daily Values (%DV) helps you gauge the nutritional value of a food item in the context of your daily diet. Values less than 5% indicate a low contribution to your daily intake, while those above 20% are considered high. If you aim to limit added sugars and unhealthy fats, avoid foods high in %DV for these nutrients. Conversely, look for higher values of fiber, vitamins, and minerals, which are beneficial for overall health (U.S. Food and Drug Administration, 2022).

Some might find it helpful to use smartphone apps designed to scan food labels and provide a quick snapshot of the product's nutritional value. These tools can be invaluable for those new to scrutinizing food labels or anyone short on time. They can offer immediate insight into whether a product aligns with your dietary goals, making your shopping experience more efficient (Katz, 2015).

Children's Foods often pose a unique challenge. Many products marketed towards kids contain excessive amounts of added sugars and unhealthy fats. Reading the labels on these products is crucial for parents wanting to set their children on a path of healthy eating. Be wary of cereals, snacks, and beverages tailored for children, as these often have hidden sugars and unhealthy fats that can contribute to long-term health issues (Moss, 2013).

Lastly, don't forget the power of whole foods—that often come without labels. Fresh fruits, vegetables, lean meats, and whole grains generally don't need an ingredient list or Nutrition Facts Panel because they are unprocessed and straightforward. Emphasizing whole foods in your diet can significantly reduce your intake of hidden sugars and unhealthy fats naturally (Pollan, 2009). But when you do opt for packaged foods, empowering yourself with the knowledge to read labels effectively can make all the difference in your journey toward better health.

In conclusion, mastering the skill of deciphering food labels will empower you to make well-informed dietary choices. This knowledge can promote overall well-being and help you align your food intake with your health goals. Always cross-check the manufacturer's claims with the Nutrition Facts Panel and ingredient list, stay wary of marketing gimmicks, and remember the added benefits of whole foods. Your health is in your hands—make it count.

Marketing to the Masses: Seeing Past the Health Hype taps into the heart of consumer decision-making. It explores how marketing tactics can mislead even the most discerning buyers. With its combination of scientific insight, motivational drive, and practical advice, this section empowers you to see beyond the health claims plastered all over food packaging.

The modern consumer is bombarded with a barrage of health claims. Every product on the shelf seems to boast about being the healthiest, the most natural, or the most beneficial for your well-being. But here's the catch: Not all these claims are as straightforward as they appear. The food industry employs an arsenal of marketing strategies designed to sell their products, often at the expense of your health (Nestle, 2013). Their goal is to make foods seem healthier than they are, masking the hidden sugars and unhealthy fats lurking within.

Marketing tactics often leverage buzzwords like "organic," "natural," or "low-fat" to sway purchasing decisions. But these terms can be misleading. For instance, a product labeled "low-fat" may indeed have reduced fat content, but it could be teeming with added sugars, enhancing flavor at the cost of your health. Understanding these marketing ploys can equip you to make informed choices, cutting through the health hype and focusing on real nutritional value.

Let's consider the "organic" label. While organic products may use fewer pesticides and be environmentally friendly, it doesn't mean they're automatically healthier from a nutritional perspective. An organic cookie still packs just as much sugar as its non-organic counterpart. The health halo around such words can make products seem more nutritious than they are, leading consumers to choose foods that don't necessarily contribute to a balanced diet (Smith-Spangler et al., 2012).

Celebrity endorsements and influential social media figures also play a significant role in shaping perceptions. When a well-known figure swears by a particular product, it doesn't automatically mean it's good for you. These endorsements are often more about marketing dollars than genuine health benefits. Remember, the ultimate aim of marketing is to sell, not necessarily to inform or educate.

To see past the health hype, it's essential to develop a critical eye. Start by scrutinizing ingredient lists and nutrition labels. Marketing messages might tell you one thing, but the fine print tells the whole story. If a product claims to be free of one harmful ingredient, check what it has as replacements. Often, manufacturers swap out one problematic component for another equally concerning one. It's a shell game where your health is at stake.

The notion of "superfoods" is another marketing marvel. While foods like avocados, blueberries, and quinoa are indeed nutritious, they're not magic bullets. Consuming superfoods in isolation won't counteract a generally poor diet or lifestyle. Balance and variety are the keys to long-term health, not the sporadic inclusion of trendy ingredients.

This leads us to another pervasive issue: front-of-package labels. Designed to catch your eye, these labels can sometimes lead you astray. Terms like "no added sugars," "whole grain," or "rich in omega-3" might give the impression of a health bonanza inside the package, but it's crucial to read the full nutrition label. "No added sugar" could still mean the product is high in natural sugars, and "whole grain" might disguise a product that is, overall, not very nutritious.

Another masterstroke of marketing is packaging design, often swathed in earthy tones and natural imagery to evoke a sense of wholesomeness. But don't be fooled by appearances. A beautiful package can conceal a multitude of unhealthy ingredients. Instead, look to food products in their most natural, unprocessed forms for your diet staples. Whole fruits, vegetables, unprocessed grains, and healthy fats are less likely to deceive you with hidden additives.

One particularly sneaky marketing tactic is the rebranding of sugar under various names. High-fructose corn syrup, cane juice, agave nectar, and myriad other aliases can appear on ingredient lists, contributing to your sugar intake without you even realizing it. The average consumer may struggle to identify all these hidden sources, but recognizing the most common sugar pseudonyms can significantly affect your dietary choices (Lustig et al., 2012).

Media influence can't be overlooked. Health-related trends are often perpetuated by popular media outlets favoring sensational headlines over accurate information. These stories can create food fads that don't always stand up to scientific scrutiny. Carb-phobia, fat aversion, and anti-gluten movements often gain traction despite limited or misrepresented scientific backing. Staying informed through reputable, science-based sources can buffer you against the constant flux of diet trends.

Educational initiatives and transparent labeling laws are steps in the right direction, but personal vigilance remains paramount. Equip yourself with reliable knowledge about nutrition, and don't hesitate to question marketing claims. By becoming a more informed consumer, you reclaim control over your health, making choices based on facts rather than easily-dismissible marketing ploys.

In conclusion, while the marketplace is awash with health claims and marketing rhetoric, your best defense is knowledge. Educate yourself on what those labels really mean, scrutinize ingredient lists, and seek out whole, minimally processed foods. This proactive approach ensures you're nourishing your body with real food, fostering lifelong wellness. Through critical thinking and informed choices, you can navigate past the health hype and toward a genuinely healthier lifestyle.

Chapter 9:
Navigating the Supermarket: Smart Shopping for Whole Foods

When stepping into a supermarket with a goal of prioritizing whole foods, a strategic approach can be your best ally. First, focus on navigating the perimeter, where fresh produce, lean meats, and dairy generally reside. These sections house most of the unprocessed, nutritious options your body naturally craves (Monaco et al., 2019). Inside aisles can be deceptive, packed with processed and sugar-laden products that compromise your health. Equip yourself with knowledge—instead of blindly trusting flashy food marketing, get familiar with reading labels critically. Look for items with a shortlist of recognizable ingredients, and skip those teeming with added sugars and unhealthy oils (Moss & Gately, 2021). Conscious, informed choices in the supermarket can significantly influence your overall wellness, helping you dodge the pitfalls of modern dietary challenges and embrace a more wholesome, nourishing lifestyle.

Strategies for Choosing Whole Over Processed are vital for anyone aiming to lead a more health-conscious lifestyle. This chapter continues our journey through "Navigating the Supermarket: Smart Shopping for Whole Foods" by presenting practical and evidence-based strategies to help you prioritize whole foods over processed ones. The goal here is to arm you with actionable insights, backed by science, to make smarter choices when you shop, thereby steering clear of the pitfalls associated with sugar and processed oils.

One straightforward strategy for choosing whole foods is to stick to the perimeter of the supermarket. Items found along the outer edges, such as fresh fruits, vegetables, meats, and dairy products, are less likely to be processed compared to those located in the center aisles. This method, sometimes referred to as "the perimeter plan," can significantly reduce the risk of picking up products laden with added sugars, oils, and other unhealthy additives (Geurts & Wendel-Vos, 2018).

Reading food labels is another critical practice. Many processed foods often contain hidden sugars, unhealthy fats, and preservatives. By spending a few extra minutes examining labels, you're better equipped to identify items with fewer ingredients, especially those you can easily recognize and pronounce. For example, if a granola bar lists ingredients like oats, nuts, and honey, it's likely a better option than one with high-fructose corn syrup, hydrogenated oils, or synthetic additives (Lustig et al., 2012). Remember, simplicity and transparency indicate fewer chances of encountering harmful ingredients.

In addition to label scrutiny, opt for foods that are as close to their natural state as possible. Fresh and frozen fruits and vegetables are fantastic choices because they tend to retain most of their nutritional value without added substances. Processed foods, on the other hand, often lose valuable nutrients during manufacturing and may compensate for this loss with artificial vitamins and minerals, which don't always offer the same health benefits (Monteiro et al., 2019).

Shopping in local farmers' markets can also be a game-changer. Produce from these markets is usually grown locally and is fresher and more nutrient-dense than items that have traveled long distances. Moreover, you're supporting sustainable practices and local economies. Consider creating a list of items you need, so you remain focused on whole food selections like fresh fruits, vegetables, lean meats, and whole grains (Jensen et al., 2019).

Preparing a meal plan in advance can majorly impact your grocery shopping habits. A well-thought-out meal plan ensures that you buy only what you need, avoiding random purchases of processed foods. Start by planning meals around seasonal fruits and vegetables, lean proteins, and whole grains. For instance, a week's meal plan could include oatmeal with fresh berries for breakfast, a salad with grilled chicken for lunch, and a sautéed vegetable stir-fry for dinner. This approach naturally minimizes the incorporation of processed foods into your diet.

Another effective strategy is cooking at home whenever possible. Dining out and relying on take-out often lead to consuming processed foods high in sugar and unhealthy fats. Cooking at home gives you complete control over ingredients and preparation methods. Simple swaps, like using olive oil instead of margarine and honey instead of refined sugars, can significantly improve your meals' nutritional quality. Over time, developing this habit can transition your entire dietary pattern towards healthier, whole food options.

Education is key. Understanding the long-term impacts of consuming processed ingredients can motivate healthier choices. For instance, high sugar intake is linked to diabetes, obesity, and cardiovascular diseases, while processed oils have been associated with inflammation and chronic conditions (Micha & Mozaffarian, 2010). Knowing these facts empowers you to make conscious decisions, leading to better health outcomes.

Motivating change can be challenging but think of it as a journey towards better health. Start with small, manageable steps. Perhaps swap out one processed snack for a whole food alternative each week. Gradually, these small changes accumulate, leading to a significant lifestyle transformation. Remember, the goal is not to strive for perfection but to make consistent improvements.

In addition, consider joining or forming a support group. Having a community of like-minded individuals can provide moral support and share practical tips for integrating whole foods into your diet. This group can also act as a sounding board for your challenges and successes, making the transition smoother and more enjoyable.

Finally, it's essential to remain flexible and compassionate with yourself. Lifestyle changes don't happen overnight, and there may be slip-ups along the way. The key is to not let these moments derail your progress. Instead, acknowledge them, understand what triggered them, and use that knowledge to make better choices in the future. After all, the journey to better health is a marathon, not a sprint.

Taking these strategies to heart can profoundly transform your shopping habits, diet, and overall well-being. As you navigate the supermarket and make more informed choices, you're not just filling your cart but investing in your health and future. Replacing processed foods with whole foods equips your body with the nutrients it needs to thrive and combat chronic diseases.

Online Review Request for This Book

If you found these strategies helpful and are noticing positive changes in your lifestyle, we'd love to hear about it! Your honest reviews can help others in their journey toward better health. Consider sharing your experiences with this book online, so we can reach and inspire more individuals aiming to make healthier choices. Thank you for being a part of this transformative journey!

The Perimeter Plan: Sticking to the Grocery Store's Outer Edges adheres to the key principle of navigating the supermarket with the aim of smart shopping for whole foods. By consciously choosing to shop along the perimeter of the grocery store, you're making a committed effort to avoid the highly processed items that dominate the center aisles. This strategy not only fosters healthier choices but also simplifies your shopping experience, making it easier to locate whole, nutrient-dense foods.

The outer edges of supermarkets are typically home to fresh produce, dairy, meat, and seafood. These sections are your allies in creating a diet rich in essential nutrients, vitamins, and minerals, without the added sugars and unhealthy fats found in processed foods. For instance, the produce section offers an array of colorful fruits and vegetables brimming with antioxidants and fiber, both crucial for maintaining a healthy digestive system and reducing the risk of chronic diseases (Slavin, 2005).

Next, the dairy aisle brings you high-quality sources of calcium and probiotics. Whether you choose milk, yogurt, or cheese, opting for products with minimal ingredients helps you stay away from unnecessary additives and sugars. Evidence shows that dairy products can play a role in improving gut health and bone density (Huth et al., 2006). However, always read the labels to avoid those sneaky sugars that like to hide even in seemingly healthy dairy options.

The meat and seafood areas also offer a bounty of protein-rich foods critical for muscle repair and overall health. When choosing your proteins, go for lean cuts and wild-caught varieties as much as possible. These selections provide a balanced intake of essential amino acids and healthy fats while avoiding the excessive sodium and preservatives found in processed meats. Quality protein is fundamental for anyone aiming to build or maintain muscle mass, including fitness enthusiasts and individuals recovering from illness (Tipton & Wolfe, 2001).

It's worth noting that while the perimeter provides many whole food options, not everything in these sections is automatically a healthy choice. For example, pre-marinated meats or fruit cups in syrup can still contain unwanted additives. Vigilance remains key. Reading labels and being aware of ingredient lists continue to be crucial practices even in these outer sections.

This shopping method aligns perfectly with our understanding of how whole foods can act as a natural antidote to processed ingredients. While the central aisles of the store are often stocked with shelves of packaged goods filled with refined sugars and unhealthy fats, sticking to the store's perimeter helps you steer clear of these pitfalls, making it easier to craft meals that nourish the body and mind. Studies have consistently shown that diets rich in whole foods are associated with lower risks of chronic conditions like heart disease, diabetes, and obesity (Liu et al., 2000).

Parents shopping for their families will find the Perimeter Plan particularly beneficial. Children's nutrition critically impacts their development and long-term health, and the outer sections of the grocery store hold the key. Fresh fruits, vegetables, dairy, meats, and whole grains support growing bodies far better than ultra-processed snacks and sugary treats. When you fill your cart with whole foods, you're setting your children up for a healthy future free from the burdens of processed food-related ailments.

Healthcare professionals and educators, too, can emphasize the importance of this shopping strategy in their guidance and teachings. Empowering patients and students with practical, actionable advice like the Perimeter Plan makes the daunting task of dietary change much more approachable. When understood and applied correctly, this method can form the foundation of long-lasting, positive dietary habits.

Fitness enthusiasts will also find the Perimeter Plan aligns with their goals. Whole foods are nutrient-dense, providing the necessary fuel for physical performance and recovery. Fresh produce supplies valuable vitamins and antioxidants, while lean proteins and dairy products offer high-quality amino acids for muscle repair and immune function. This approach helps maintain energy levels and supports overall health, leading to better workout outcomes and muscle regeneration (Phillips & Van Loon, 2011).

Before concluding this section, we need to remind ourselves of the principles underpinning the Perimeter Plan. The ultimate goal is to simplify healthy eating by returning to basics. Instead of being overwhelmed by the myriad of food choices, focusing on whole, unprocessed items found in the periphery of the supermarket streamlines your shopping experience. It's a user-friendly strategy that can have profound impacts on your health and well-being.

Adopting this approach means you're taking charge of your diet, actively choosing foods that contribute to longevity and vitality. The Perimeter Plan can transform your relationship with food, empowering you to make informed choices that benefit every aspect of your life. Remember, the journey to a healthier lifestyle begins with each trip to the grocery store. Stick to the edges, and you're already halfway there to achieving your health goals.

As you implement the Perimeter Plan in your own shopping habits, consider the ripple effects. Each purchase you make supports a market for healthier food options, potentially influencing broader dietary trends. This collective shift can create a demand for better quality foods and prompt changes in how supermarkets stock their shelves, fostering a healthier society at large.

In conclusion, **The Perimeter Plan: Sticking to the Grocery Store's Outer Edges** offers a straightforward yet highly effective method for navigating the supermarket with an eye towards health. By concentrating your shopping efforts on the outer sections of the store, you naturally gravitate towards nutrient-rich, whole foods that support a balanced, healthy diet. This strategy not only simplifies your grocery shopping but also lays the groundwork for lasting health improvements, making it easier for individuals and families alike to make better food choices every day.

Chapter 10:
The Power of Whole Foods: Nature's Antidote to Processed Ingredients

The Power of Whole Foods: Nature's Antidote to Processed Ingredients lies in their unparalleled ability to nourish the body and mind, providing essential nutrients that are often stripped away in their processed counterparts. From vibrant fruits and vegetables to nutrient-dense grains and lean proteins, whole foods are nature's pharmacy, offering an array of vitamins, minerals, and antioxidants that work synergistically to support our health. Scientific evidence has consistently demonstrated that diets rich in whole foods can reduce the risk of chronic diseases such as heart disease, diabetes, and obesity (Micha et al., 2017; Mozaffarian et al., 2018). Moreover, these foods are digested more slowly than processed foods, leading to more stable blood sugar levels and sustained energy throughout the day (Ludwig, 2002). In embracing a diet centered around whole foods, we empower ourselves with the tools to combat the damaging effects of processed ingredients, fostering both physical resilience and mental clarity.

The Benefits of a Whole Foods Diet provide a compelling counterpoint to the proliferation of processed ingredients in modern diets. When we talk about whole foods, we're referring to foods that are minimally processed and remain as close to their natural state as possible. Think fruits, vegetables, whole grains, nuts, seeds, and lean proteins. These are the building blocks for a diet that not only nourishes but also fosters long-term health and well-being.

Why are whole foods so beneficial? One of the main reasons is their nutrient density. Unlike their processed counterparts, whole foods are rich in essential vitamins, minerals, and phytonutrients that our bodies need to function optimally. For example, a simple apple offers fiber, vitamin C, and a range of antioxidants, all of which work together to support immune function and digestive health (Liu, 2003). On the other hand, a processed apple snack might lose much of these nutrients through the manufacturing process, leaving behind empty calories.

Moreover, whole foods promote better digestion thanks to their high fiber content. Fiber is crucial for maintaining a healthy gut, which in turn influences everything from nutrient absorption to mood regulation. A diet rich in whole foods helps ensure that the gut microbiome—the community of bacteria and other microorganisms living in the digestive tract—remains balanced and healthy. Research indicates that a diverse microbiome can lower the risk of chronic diseases, including obesity and type 2 diabetes (Sonnenburg & Sonnenburg, 2014).

Consuming whole foods can also help manage weight more effectively. Whole foods are generally lower in calories yet higher in satiety compared to processed foods. This means you're less likely to overeat when your diet consists primarily of whole foods. For instance, eating a bowl of oatmeal made from whole oats can keep you full and energized much longer than consuming a bowl of sugary cereal. The fiber in the oatmeal slows digestion, promoting sustained energy release and helping you avoid the spikes and crashes often associated with processed carbs (Slavin, 2005).

An often overlooked benefit is the positive impact on mental health. Emerging research shows that diets high in whole foods are linked to lower rates of depression and anxiety. Nutrients like omega-3 fatty acids, found in foods such as fatty fish and flaxseeds, have been shown to play a role in brain health and mood regulation (Bodnar & Wisner, 2005). Additionally, complex carbohydrates from whole grains can stabilize blood sugar levels, providing a steady stream of energy to the brain and reducing the mood swings that can come from eating processed sugars.

Whole foods also shine in disease prevention and management. The antioxidants and anti-inflammatory compounds found in fruits and vegetables help combat oxidative stress, which has been linked to a variety of chronic illnesses including heart disease, cancer, and Alzheimer's (Liu, 2003). For instance, the lycopene in tomatoes and the sulforaphane in broccoli are both potent compounds known for their disease-fighting properties.

Another significant advantage is that a whole foods diet supports environmental sustainability. Foods that are minimally processed generally require fewer resources to produce and are often less taxing on the environment. Opting for whole foods typically means choosing items that are less packaged and processed, circumventing the harmful cycle of waste and pollution associated with the production and disposal of processed food items (Robertson, 2014).

This all ties back to the overall aim of our book, which is to educate and empower you to make healthier dietary choices. Understanding the benefits of whole foods isn't just academic; it's practical. The more you know about what these foods can do for you, the more motivated you'll be to incorporate them into your daily life.

In our section on reading between the labels, we discussed how to spot hidden sugars and unhealthy oils. Another critical skill is recognizing whole foods in their purest forms. Fruits without added sugars, vegetables without preservatives, and grains that haven't been stripped of their nutrients are invaluable. Making a concerted effort to focus on these whole, unaltered ingredients can set the stage for a healthier, more vibrant you.

For those navigating the often confusing aisles of supermarkets, prioritizing whole foods can simplify your shopping. Sticking to the perimeter of the store, where fresh produce, dairy, and meats are usually found, can help you avoid the pitfalls of processed convenience foods. This strategy not only ensures you're more likely to pick nutrient-dense options but can also be more economical in the long run. Whole foods often cost less per serving than processed options when nutrients and satiety are taken into account (Carlson & Frazão, 2014).

Now, when we consider the impact of a whole foods diet on children, the benefits are even more striking. Developing bodies and brains need a steady supply of nutrients to grow optimally. Whole foods provide that essential nutrition without the additives and preservatives that might negatively impact their development. Encouraging children to enjoy whole foods from an early age can set up healthy eating patterns that last a lifetime, possibly lowering their risk of chronic illnesses later in life (Ventura & Birch, 2008).

Putting these principles into practice may seem daunting, but it doesn't have to be. Simple steps like meal planning, cooking in bulk, and packing nutrient-dense snacks can ease the transition. From experience, once you start feeling the advantages—more energy, better digestion, improved mood—it becomes a positive feedback loop. You'll see firsthand how nourishing your body with whole foods pays off, making it easier to stay committed to this lifestyle.

In essence, a whole foods diet isn't just a passing trend; it's a return to basics, to what our bodies have evolved to thrive on. It's an antidote to the processed ingredients that have come to dominate modern diets. By cutting down on refined sugars and unhealthy fats while embracing the variety and richness of whole foods, we don't just eat better—we live better.

Your journey to a healthier you may start with understanding the risks associated with processed foods, but it finds its fulfillment in the abundant benefits of whole foods. By making mindful choices and focusing on natural, unprocessed ingredients, you safeguard not only your health but also the health of future generations.

For those motivated to take the next step, consider this an invitation to dive deeper. The upcoming chapters will provide actionable tips on how to replace sugars and oils in your recipes, strategies for smart shopping, and even meal planning guides. Integrating whole foods into your lifestyle is not a one-size-fits-all approach, but it's an adventure well worth embarking on, filled with opportunities for growth, learning, and lasting well-being.

By understanding and embracing the benefits of a whole foods diet, you're setting up a foundation for a lifetime of health and vitality. As you explore these nutritional fundamentals, you'll discover how whole foods can transform not just your diet, but your overall quality of life.

Online Review Request for This Book If you've found value in the insights and research shared in this book, we kindly ask you to take a moment to leave an online review. Your feedback helps

Satisfying Sweetness: Natural Sugar Alternatives invites readers to explore the delightful universe of natural sweeteners, offering a path to joyous consumption without sacrificing health. We live in a time where the adverse effects of refined sugar are becoming increasingly evident, linked to a myriad of health issues such as obesity, diabetes, and heart disease (Johnson et al., 2009). As people become more health-conscious, the demand for healthier alternatives is now higher than ever. Fortunately, nature, in its bounty, offers a variety of delightful options that can satisfy our sweet tooth without compromising our well-being.

Sweet and Slick

One of the most popular natural sweeteners is stevia, derived from the leaves of the Stevia rebaudiana plant. Stevia has been celebrated for quite some time in South America, but it's recently gained worldwide popularity due to its zero-calorie content and its capacity to be up to 300 times sweeter than sugar (Chatsudthipong & Muanprasat, 2009). This makes it an excellent choice for those looking to manage weight and maintain stable blood sugar levels. Another benefit? Unlike artificial sweeteners, stevia is entirely natural, offering an appealing option not just for individuals with specific dietary needs, but for anyone seeking a more natural diet.

Next on the list is honey, which isn't merely a sweet nectar but a nutrient-rich powerhouse. Raw honey contains vitamins, antioxidants, and enzymes that offer a range of health benefits, from soothing sore throats to providing a burst of natural energy (Bogdanov et al., 2008). However, it is essential to note that honey is still high in fructose and should be consumed in moderation. It's not a free pass to indulge but rather a means to enjoy sweetness more responsibly.

For those who appreciate culinary diversity, maple syrup is another excellent option. Harvested from the sap of maple trees, this syrup is not only delicious but also rich in minerals like manganese and zinc. These nutrients are essential for bone health and immune function (Moser et al., 2015). When choosing maple syrup, it's best to opt for the pure, organic varieties to avoid added sugars and preservatives typically found in commercial brands. A drizzle of this golden delight can elevate anything from pancakes to roasted vegetables without the guilt associated with refined sugars.

Date sugar, made from finely ground dried dates, is another natural sweetener growing in popularity. Apart from providing a rich, caramel-like flavor, dates are high in fiber, antioxidants, and various vitamins and minerals. They offer a much-needed break from the empty calories of refined sugars, adding nutritional value to your diet

(Al-Farsi & Lee, 2008). Since date sugar doesn't dissolve well in liquids, it's perfect for baking and can be a delightful enhancement for your favorite recipes.

Coconut sugar, derived from the sap of the coconut palm, is a low-glycemic sweetener, making it a viable option for those managing blood sugar issues (Arumughan et al., 2009). Rich in vitamins and minerals, including iron, zinc, potassium, and calcium, coconut sugar also contains inulin, a type of fiber that acts as a prebiotic and promotes gut health. The subtly caramel flavor of coconut sugar makes it an excellent substitute in recipes calling for brown sugar or similar sweeteners.

Beyond these well-known options, one must not forget about monk fruit sweetener. Extracted from the monk fruit or Luo Han Guo, this sweetener is incredibly potent, rated up to 250 times sweeter than sugar while being calorie-free. What makes monk fruit especially unique is its antioxidant properties, which have been shown to offer numerous health benefits including anti-inflammatory and anti-carcinogenic effects (Di et al., 2011). This sweetener is becoming more accessible and is a great addition to the toolkit of anyone looking to reduce their sugar intake.

Each of these natural alternatives provides a better option for maintaining sweetness in our diets while promoting better health. It's critical, however, to remember that even natural sweeteners should be used thoughtfully. Moderation remains the key. These alternatives can undoubtedly provide a healthier path, yet indulging in excessive quantities can still lead to health issues. It's all about finding the right balance and making informed choices.

As we've explored these natural sweeteners, remember their integration goes beyond just replacing sugar; it's about adopting a lifestyle where whole foods become the cornerstone of your diet. Whole foods, as nature intended, offer a more refined approach to nutrition that goes hand-in-hand with mindful living. They allow you to enjoy the foods you love without the hidden pitfalls of processed ingredients that plague modern diets. Embracing natural sweeteners is but one step towards a more holistic approach to nutrition.

When considering lifestyle changes, especially in terms of diet, remember that science and personal health have to walk hand in hand. Natural sugar alternatives not only offer their nutritional benefits but also play a role in societal trends towards more sustainable and health-conscious living. They provide a way to indulge in the comfort of sweetness while contributing positively to long-term health outcomes.

In your journey towards a healthier you, these natural sugar alternatives can serve as beacons of hope, lighting the way towards a diet that is both satisfying and nutritious. Whether you're a parent aiming to set a better example for your children, a health-conscious individual, or a healthcare professional providing guidance, these alternatives can make a significant difference. By embracing them, we can take a stand against the tide of processed ingredients that have inundated our diets and take a step towards a more vibrant, health-conscious future.

Ultimately, the power of choice lies in your hands. The allure of sweetness does not have to come at the cost of your well-being. Through educated and informed decisions, it's entirely possible to maintain a satisfying level of sweetness in your diet while prioritizing long-term health. In the context of our broader journey through whole foods, these natural sugar alternatives offer not just a way to sweeten our foods, but a sweeter path to a healthier life.

Chapter 11:
From Kitchen to Table: Cooking with Whole Ingredients

Cooking with whole ingredients transforms not just meals but entire lifestyles, bridging the gap between healthful intentions and practical implementation. Imagine trading processed sugars and oils for their natural counterparts—honey instead of high-fructose corn syrup, olive oil over hydrogenated fats. Such changes may seem small but yield significant health benefits, helping to reduce inflammation, improve cardiovascular health, and manage weight effectively (Hu et al., 2019). Mastering techniques like steaming, roasting, and fermenting can elevate the nutritional profile of food while preserving its intrinsic flavors. Practical strategies, such as using spices and herbs for seasoning instead of sugar-laden sauces, empower families to enjoy food that's both delicious and healthful. Through mindful preparation and ingredient selection, you can create meals that provide nourishment and joy, fostering a holistic sense of well-being for yourself and loved ones.

The Art of Healthful Cooking: Techniques and Tips often starts with a deep understanding of the ingredients you're working with. Cooking with whole ingredients isn't just a trend; it's a journey towards embracing a healthier lifestyle.

One of the most powerful techniques for healthful cooking is mastering the art of substitution. By replacing refined sugars and processed oils with natural alternatives, you can make your meals both nutritious and delicious. For example, using honey or maple syrup instead of refined white sugar not only adds sweetness but also contributes nutrients like antioxidants and minerals (Nutritional Review, 2017). Similarly, opting for extra virgin olive oil instead of margarine or corn oil can improve the flavor of your dishes while delivering heart-healthy monounsaturated fats (Estruch et al., 2018).

However, it's not just about swapping ingredients; it's also about techniques that retain the nutrients and enhance the flavors of the natural foods. One method is steaming, which can be particularly beneficial for vegetables. Steaming preserves the vitamins and minerals that might otherwise be lost in the cooking water, giving you a more nutritious meal. Sautéing with a small amount of healthy oil like avocado oil is another great technique. It allows you to bring out the vibrant colors and flavors of your ingredients without overwhelming them with unhealthy fats.

Let's talk about herbs and spices. These natural flavor enhancers can turn a simple dish into a culinary masterpiece while providing a slew of health benefits. For instance, turmeric, known for its anti-inflammatory properties, can be added to soups, stews, and even smoothies. Fresh herbs like basil, cilantro, and parsley not only provide vibrant green hues but also offer a plethora of vitamins and antioxidants (Aggarwal & Sung, 2009). Using these herbs and spices allows you to reduce the amount of salt and fat in your recipes without compromising on flavor.

Another invaluable tip for healthful cooking is to focus on cooking methods that minimize the addition of unnecessary fats. Techniques like grilling, broiling, and roasting can impart a delicious, smoky flavor to meats and vegetables without the need for additional oils. When roasting, using a parchment paper can reduce the need for greasing your baking sheets. This not only makes for easy cleanup but also keeps your dishes lower in calories.

A common pitfall in healthful cooking is overlooking the impact of portion sizes. Even when cooking with whole ingredients, portion control is crucial. Using smaller plates and serving utensils can naturally reduce the amount of food and, consequently, the calories you consume. Additionally, integrating more abundant vegetables and whole grains like quinoa and brown rice can help you feel fuller longer, reducing the temptation to overeat.

Moreover, mindful cooking practices can elevate the healthfulness of your meals. Taking the time to plan and prepare your meals can reduce the reliance on convenience foods, which often contain added sugars and unhealthy fats. Batch cooking is a great strategy for busy individuals and families. Preparing large quantities of whole foods and storing them in portioned containers can make it easier to maintain a nutritious diet throughout the week.

Online Review Request for This Book: "The Art of Healthful Cooking: Techniques and Tips" concludes with a gentle reminder to our readers to share their experience with this book. Your thoughts and reviews can be the beacon of encouragement for others to embark on this journey to a healthier lifestyle. If you found the insights and strategies valuable, please take a moment to leave a review online. Your feedback not only supports our mission to spread knowledge about the impact of sugar and processed oils on health but also empowers others to make life-changing dietary choices. Thank you for contributing to a healthier future!

Small Swaps, Big Impact: Replacing Sugars and Oils in Recipes is about making minor changes in our cooking habits that can have profound effects on our overall health. In other words, you don't need to overhaul your diet overnight; even slight modifications can help steer you toward a healthier lifestyle. Let's dive into practical ways to replace conventional sugars and processed oils in your favorite recipes without sacrificing flavor or texture. These swaps are not only feasible but can bring significant long-term benefits, particularly for those conscious of conditions such as diabetes, heart disease, and inflammatory disorders.

Consider your morning cup of coffee or tea. While a teaspoon of sugar may seem harmless, it adds up over the course of a day, month, or year. An easy swap? Try stevia, a natural sweetener derived from the Stevia rebaudiana plant. Stevia contains no calories and has little to no impact on blood sugar levels (Lohner et al., 2017). It's a small change but can substantially reduce your daily sugar intake.

When it comes to baked goods, like muffins or cookies, applesauce and mashed bananas make excellent substitutes for sugar. These natural sweeteners not only cut down on pure sugar but also add a dose of vitamins, minerals, and fiber. A good rule of thumb is to use half a cup of puréed fruit for every cup of sugar the recipe calls for. Keep in mind that this might slightly alter the moisture content of the final product, so slight adjustments may be necessary.

And what about oils? Processed vegetable oils like canola, sunflower, and safflower are a common sight in many kitchens. Unfortunately, these oils are often high in omega-6 fatty acids, which, when consumed in excess, can contribute to inflammation and chronic disease (Simopoulos, 2002). Instead, consider using extra virgin olive oil or coconut oil. These fats are more stable at higher cooking temperatures and boast a range of health benefits.

Extra virgin olive oil is rich in monounsaturated fats, which have been shown to improve heart health by reducing bad cholesterol levels and increasing good cholesterol (Pérez-Jiménez & Ruano, 2001). Use it for sautéing vegetables or as a base for homemade salad dressings.

Coconut oil, on the other hand, is rich in medium-chain triglycerides (MCTs), which can boost metabolism and energy levels (St-Onge & Bosarge, 2008). It is particularly good in baking and can even replace butter in some recipes. However, it's essential to use unrefined, virgin coconut oil to avoid added chemicals and preservatives.

For those who enjoy the texture and flavor of butter in their recipes, consider using ghee, a form of clarified butter that removes milk solids and water, leaving behind a more concentrated, buttery fat. Ghee has a higher smoke point than regular butter and is rich in fat-soluble vitamins like A, D, and E (Gurr, 1992).

Let's not forget the role of spices and herbs in creating flavorful dishes that rely less on added sugars and oils. Cinnamon, for example, can add a natural sweetness to dishes without the need for sugar. It's perfect for oatmeal, smoothies, and baked goods. Similarly, herbs like rosemary, thyme, and basil can enhance the flavor profile of a dish, allowing you to use less oil for taste.

Blend healthier cooking practices into your routine slowly. Instead of feeling overwhelmed by the magnitude of dietary changes, make one or two swaps per week. Over time, these small changes will accumulate, yielding significant health benefits without feeling restricting or unattainable. Remember, change doesn't need to be dramatic to be effective.

Are you ready to make a change? Consider documenting your journey. Track your swaps and their impacts on your health and well-being. Share your experiences in an online review for this book. Not only will it help others who are on a similar journey, but it can also serve as a motivational tool for you. Knowing that your actions are making a difference can provide the emotional reinforcement needed to stick with new habits.

As you experiment with these alternative ingredients, you may find that you begin to appreciate the nuanced flavors natural foods can offer. This can create a more enjoyable and sustainable approach to healthy eating, one that you're more likely to stick with in the long run.

Finally, it's crucial to remain informed and continually seek knowledge. Science continually evolves, and being up-to-date with the latest research can empower you to make the best choices for your health. Take note of how your body responds to these changes and adjust accordingly. After all, the ultimate goal is to find what works best for you and your unique needs.

By making these small swaps, and sharing your experiences through an online review of this book, you're not just making a difference in your own life. You're contributing to a larger movement towards healthier, more sustainable dietary habits for everyone.

Chapter 12:
Creating a Sustainable Diet: Long-Term Strategies for Better Health

Creating a sustainable diet is about forming a balance between immediate dietary changes and lifelong habits that support health and well-being. You don't need dramatic overhauls; start with pragmatic shifts, like balancing macronutrients (carbs, fats, and proteins) within your meals. Integrating whole foods, reducing processed sugars and oils, and setting achievable goals can lead to transformative health benefits. Research demonstrates that small, consistent changes foster long-term adherence and success (Ludwig & Ebbeling, 2018). By harnessing the power of informed food choices and gradual lifestyle adjustments, everyone—from parents shaping their children's diets to fitness enthusiasts optimizing performance—can work toward a healthier future (Mozaffarian et al., 2019).

Balancing Macronutrients: A Harmony of Carbs, Fats, and Proteins plays a pivotal role in creating a sustainable diet. By striking the right balance between carbohydrates, fats, and proteins, we can set the stage for optimal health, stable energy levels, and well-rounded nutrition. A harmonious diet isn't just about the foods we choose; it's about understanding how these macronutrients work together to support our bodies' functions and long-term vitality.

When we talk about balanced macronutrients, we often start with carbohydrates. Carbs are the body's primary energy source. However, not all carbs are created equal. Complex carbohydrates, like those found in whole grains, vegetables, and legumes, provide sustained energy and are rich in fiber, which improves digestive health. On the flip side, simple carbohydrates, such as those in sugary snacks and sodas, can cause spikes in blood sugar levels and lead to energy crashes afterward (Ludwig, 2002).

Fats are another crucial component of a balanced diet. They are essential for brain health, hormone production, and the absorption of fat-soluble vitamins (vitamins A, D, E, and K). Emphasizing healthy forms of fat, such as monounsaturated and polyunsaturated fatty acids, is key. These healthy fats can be found in foods like avocados, nuts, seeds, and fatty fish. Conversely, limiting trans fats and hydrogenated oils, often found in fried and processed foods, can reduce the risk of chronic diseases such as heart disease (Mozaffarian et al., 2006).

Proteins are the building blocks of our body tissues and play a vital role in muscle repair, immune function, and the production of enzymes and hormones. Both plant-based and animal-based proteins have essential roles, and finding the right mix can contribute to a balanced, sustainable diet. Sources like lean meats, dairy, beans, and lentils offer a variety of nutrients beyond just protein. Diversifying protein sources also ensures an adequate intake of essential amino acids necessary for overall health (Rodriguez, 2015).

One of the biggest challenges in balancing macronutrients is understanding individual needs and preferences. Factors such as age, gender, activity level, and specific health conditions can influence the ideal ratio of carbs, fats, and proteins. This is where personalized nutrition plans become invaluable. By tailoring macronutrient intake to our unique biological and lifestyle requirements, we can optimize our diets for better health outcomes.

Now, let's consider how balancing these macronutrients creates a harmonious diet. Imagine a diet that is too high in carbohydrates but low in fats and proteins; this could lead to rapid energy fluctuations and potential nutrient deficiencies. Conversely, a diet too high in fats without adequate carbohydrates or proteins can result in suboptimal energy levels and impede muscle repair and growth. Striking a balance ensures that our energy levels remain steady, our muscles and tissues repair efficiently, and our bodies function optimally (Paddon-Jones et al., 2009).

The art of balancing macronutrients goes hand-in-hand with meal planning and mindful eating. Planning meals that incorporate a variety of macronutrient-rich foods can help achieve the right balance. For example, a well-rounded breakfast could include whole-grain toast (carbs), avocado (fats), and eggs (proteins). This combination provides prolonged energy, supports brain function, and helps with muscle repair from the get-go.

Additionally, being mindful of portion sizes is crucial. Overeating any macronutrient can lead to an excess caloric intake, which may result in weight gain and associated health issues. By understanding the importance of each macronutrient and their recommended daily intakes, we can make informed choices that support our health goals. Tools like food journals or nutrition tracking apps can aid in this effort, making it easier to visualize and adjust our macronutrient intake as needed.

Balancing macronutrients also has significant benefits for managing specific health conditions. For individuals with diabetes, maintaining balanced carbohydrate intake is critical for controlling blood sugar levels. Including healthy fats and proteins in meals can moderate the absorption of glucose, preventing sudden spikes and dips in blood sugar (Hu et al., 2001). Similarly, individuals with cardiovascular concerns may find that emphasizing healthy fats and reducing processed carbohydrates can improve lipid profiles and overall heart health.

What about the interplay between macronutrients and exercise? For fitness enthusiasts and athletes, the timing and composition of macronutrient intake can greatly influence performance and recovery. Carbs play a pivotal role in replenishing glycogen stores post-exercise, while proteins are essential for muscle repair and growth. Healthy fats can aid in reducing inflammation and supporting long-term energy needs. By understanding these dynamics, athletes can optimize their diets to enhance their performance and recovery cycle (Louise et al., 2019).

It's also essential to recognize that cultural and personal food preferences play a role in balancing macronutrients. Diverse dietary patterns, whether vegetarian, vegan, Mediterranean, or others, can all achieve macronutrient balance through thoughtful food choices. Embracing this diversity allows us to make sustainable changes that align with our lifestyle and culinary preferences, making it more likely that these healthy habits will stick.

Incorporating variety within each macronutrient category is another strategy for ensuring nutrient adequacy and preventing dietary monotony. For carbohydrates, this might mean rotating between different whole grains like quinoa, brown rice, and oats. For fats, it could involve using olive oil, coconut oil, and nut butters. Meanwhile, protein diversity might include mixing plant-based proteins like beans and tofu with lean meats and dairy. This approach not only enhances nutrient intake but also keeps meals interesting and satisfying.

Lastly, education is a cornerstone of creating a balanced macronutrient strategy. Understanding the sources and roles of different macronutrients empowers us to make informed choices that support long-term health. By sharing evidence-based information and practical tips, we can inspire others to take proactive steps towards better nutrition. Healthcare professionals, educators, and community leaders all play vital roles in disseminating this knowledge and supporting individuals on their journey to balanced diets. Through collaborative efforts, we can foster a culture of health that values the interplay of carbohydrates, fats, and proteins.

As you reflect on these principles, consider how you can incorporate balanced macronutrients into your daily life. Experiment with meal planning, diversify your food choices, and stay mindful of your unique nutritional needs. Remember, the goal is to create a sustainable, enjoyable diet that supports your health and well-being in the long term. By achieving harmony in your macronutrient intake, you're taking a significant step towards a healthier, more vibrant life.

Setting Achievable Goals: Taking Steps Toward Dietary Change is the cornerstone of creating lasting and meaningful improvements in your health via dietary choices. Many have the determination to overhaul their diets, yet the challenge lies in translating this motivation into practical, daily habits. Let's delve into how you can set realistic and manageable dietary goals that serve to ensure long-term health benefits.

First and foremost, recognize that achieving transformative dietary change begins with a clear vision of what you wish to accomplish. Instead of vaguely aiming to "eat healthier," be specific about your goals. For example, you might decide to "reduce added sugar intake by half" or "replace trans fats with healthier polyunsaturated and monounsaturated fats." These precise targets are more actionable and measurable, making it easier to track progress and stay motivated.

One effective strategy is to adopt the SMART criteria when setting goals: Specific, Measurable, Achievable, Relevant, and Time-bound. For instance, a SMART goal could be: "I will reduce my weekly intake of sugary snacks from seven servings to three over the next month."

Beginning with small, incremental steps can make a world of difference. Suppose you currently consume multiple servings of processed snacks every day. An immediate and drastic reduction might be overwhelming and unsustainable. Instead, start by eliminating one or two servings per week. These small adjustments accumulate over time, gradually shifting your dietary habits without the stress of abrupt changes.

Another essential aspect is to embrace flexibility in your goals. Life is unpredictable, and adherence to dietary changes isn't always linear. Allow yourself the grace to occasionally deviate from your plan without feeling guilty or discouraged. The key is to maintain a general trajectory towards healthier eating, rather than obsessing over occasional lapses.

Explore substitutions that spirit you towards your goals without sacrificing enjoyment. For sugar reduction, consider natural sweeteners like stevia or monk fruit, which can provide sweetness with fewer negative health impacts (Rippe & Angelopoulos, 2016). Likewise, for fats, look to replace trans fats with sources of omega-3 fatty acids found in flaxseeds, chia seeds, and fish (Mozaffarian et al., 2021).

It's also important to stay informed and educated about nutrition. Many fall prey to marketing tactics that promote unhealthy foods as healthy options. Developing skills to properly read and understand food labels can empower you to make better choices. Focus on whole foods, minimal ingredient lists, and natural sources of nutrients (Nestle, 2013).

Your environment plays a pivotal role as well. If your pantry is stocked with processed foods, the temptation will always be present. Align your environment with your goals—fill your kitchen with whole foods, fruits, vegetables, nuts, and seeds. Creating a consistent, supportive environment facilitates easier adherence to your dietary objectives.

Enlisting support from family, friends, or communities can further consolidate your commitment. Sharing your goals with others makes you accountable and provides a network of encouragement, practical advice, and shared experiences. Many people find success in joining support groups or online forums dedicated to healthy eating.

Lastly, recognize and celebrate your achievements along the way. Each milestone reached is a step closer to a sustained, healthy lifestyle. Employ strategies to keep yourself motivated—whether through rewards, keeping a progress journal, or periodic self-reflection on the benefits already gained.

Real, impactful dietary change is a journey that involves patience, perseverance, and a positive mindset. Setting achievable goals forms the bedrock of this journey. As you start taking small, realistic steps toward reducing sugar and processed fats, you'll not only see improvements in your health but also establish habits that can last a lifetime.

Engage with the further sections of this book, as they will offer additional insights and practical tips to support your continued journey toward better dietary habits. Remember, each positive change you make, no matter how small, brings you one step closer to your goal of achieving a sustainable, healthful diet.

Adopting these strategies ensures you aren't just making temporary fixes, but forging a new lifestyle that champions long-term health and well-being.

Online Review Request for This Book

We genuinely appreciate your engagement with our book and hope it has been a valuable resource on your journey toward healthier dietary habits. If you found the content insightful and beneficial, we kindly request you to leave a review online. Your feedback helps us improve and assists other readers in discovering valuable resources. Thank you for your support and dedication to better health!

Online Review Request for This Book

If you found "Creating a Sustainable Diet: Long-Term Strategies for Better Health" enlightening and helpful, please consider leaving a review online to help others discover how evidence-based dietary changes can transform their health and well-being.

Chapter 13:
The Road to Health Is Paved with Sweet Intentions

As we've journeyed through the complexities of sugar and processed oils, it's clear that the path to health isn't about rigid restrictions but rather about mindful and informed choices. The road to health truly is paved with sweet intentions—intentions to prioritize our well-being, to nourish our bodies with whole foods, to educate ourselves and others, and to make sustainable changes that can enhance our quality of life.

Understanding the science behind sugar and oils is crucial. It's not enough to merely know that too much sugar or the wrong types of fats are harmful. We need to understand why and how current consumption patterns contribute to various health issues. The data we've explored reveals a stark reality: overconsumption of sugar and processed oils is linked to obesity, diabetes, heart disease, and inflammation (Smith et al., 2016). Recognizing these links empowers us to make informed decisions about what we eat.

Yet knowledge alone isn't sufficient. Motivation and practical strategies are equally vital. The principles of a whole-foods diet offer one such strategy. Embracing whole foods means moving beyond calorie counting and ingredient restrictions. It's about fostering a profound connection with what we consume. Fresh fruits, vegetables, nuts, seeds, and lean proteins aren't just nutritional necessities; they're the building blocks of a vibrant life. Opting for natural sweeteners like honey or maple syrup, and healthier fats like those found in avocados and olive oil, encourages balance and well-being (Johnson, 2007).

For parents, the intention to raise healthier children is key. Instilling good dietary habits from a young age sets the foundation for lifelong health. Children learn by example, and making conscious food choices can create a ripple effect through generations. The impact of reducing sugary snacks and processed foods can be profound, aiding in better concentration, mood stability, and long-term health (Lustig, 2013). Engaging children in meal planning and preparation can further solidify these lessons, embedding the importance of nutrition in their lives.

Healthcare professionals and educators play a unique role, too. They're at the forefront of disseminating this vital information. Whether through patient consultations, classroom teaching, or public health campaigns, professionals can ignite a broader movement toward better dietary practices. By advocating for clearer food labeling and challenging misleading marketing, they serve as catalysts for change. This societal shift toward transparency and education can have far-reaching consequences, empowering individuals to make healthful choices.

Our journey also highlights that small, incremental changes can lead to significant health improvements over time. You don't have to overhaul your diet overnight. Start by swapping out one processed snack for a piece of fruit. Replace a handful of chips with a handful of nuts. Over time, these small adjustments can become habits, and those habits can transform your health landscape. Achieving balance in our diets isn't about perfect adherence to rigid guidelines; it's about consistent, thoughtful choices that align with our sweet intentions.

Community support is another cornerstone. Sharing recipes, cooking tips, and encouragement with friends and family can create a supportive environment that nurtures collective well-being. The shared experience of trying new foods and discovering healthier alternatives can be both educational and enjoyable. Building a community around healthy eating can motivate everyone to stay committed to their health goals.

Finally, sustainability is paramount. Long-term health stems from practices that are manageable and enjoyable. Crash diets and extreme restrictions are often unsustainable and can do more harm than good. Instead, cultivating a sustainable approach to diet and lifestyle ensures that the benefits we reap are long-lasting. This includes being mindful of our environmental impact as well. Choosing locally-sourced and organic foods not only supports local businesses but also encourages sustainable farming practices, contributing to the overall health of our planet.

In conclusion, our journey through the world of sugar and processed oils has equipped us with the tools to make healthier choices. By understanding the science, leveraging practical strategies, and maintaining our sweet intentions, we can pave our own roads to better health. As you move forward, remember that every small choice counts. Each piece of fruit over a candy bar, each meal cooked at home rather than ordered out, each step is a stride toward better health. Let's commit to these intentions, for ourselves and for future generations.

Appendix A:
Further Reading and Resources

If you've made it this far, you're likely committed to making healthier choices for yourself and your loved ones. Understanding the impact of sugar and processed oils is just the beginning. To further your knowledge and equip yourself with actionable information, this appendix provides an array of resources, spanning books, academic journals, websites, and expert organizations. Dive deep into these readings and use the listed resources to continue growing on your health journey.

Books

- *Salt Sugar Fat: How the Food Giants Hooked Us* by Michael Moss - This insightful book looks at how major food corporations have manipulated ingredients to make products irresistible (Moss, 2013).

- *Good Calories, Bad Calories* by Gary Taubes - An in-depth analysis of the role of sugar and fats in diet and disease, supported by extensive research (Taubes, 2007).

- *The Big Fat Surprise: Why Butter, Meat, and Cheese Belong in a Healthy Diet* by Nina Teicholz - An investigative work revealing the flawed science behind dietary fat guidelines (Teicholz, 2014).

Academic Journals

- *American Journal of Clinical Nutrition* - A leading journal in nutrition science, providing evidence-based research on the effects of sugar and fats on health. Key articles such as "Dietary Fats and Cardiovascular Disease: A Review of the Evidence" can be found here (Astrup et al., 2021).

- *The Lancet* - Publishes high-impact medical research, including studies on dietary habits and health outcomes. Articles like "Sugar-Sweetened Beverages and Risk of Metabolic Syndrome and Type 2 Diabetes" offer valuable insights (Malik et al., 2010).

- *Journal of the American Medical Association (JAMA)* - This journal covers comprehensive health research, including dietary studies like "Association of Low-Carbohydrate and Low-Fat Diets With Mortality Among US Adults" (Seidelmann et al., 2018).

Websites and Online Resources

- **NutritionFacts.org** - Offers videos and blogs on nutrition research, focusing on evidence-based dietary advice (NutritionFacts.org, n.d.).

- **Centers for Disease Control and Prevention (CDC) - Nutrition** - This government site provides guidelines and tips for healthy eating (CDC, n.d.).

- **Mayo Clinic - Healthy Lifestyle Nutrition and Healthy Eating** - Offers expert advice and science-backed information on nutrition and dietary choices (Mayo Clinic, n.d.).

Organizations

- **American Heart Association (AHA)** - Provides guidelines and resources on heart-healthy diets with an emphasis on reducing sugar and unhealthy fats (AHA, n.d.).

- **World Health Organization (WHO)** - Global guidelines on sugar intake and recommendations for preventing chronic diseases (WHO, n.d.).

- **Academy of Nutrition and Dietetics** - Offers resources for understanding nutrition science and applying it to everyday eating habits (Academy of Nutrition and Dietetics, n.d.).

Using these resources, you can continue to explore the science behind dietary choices and their impacts on health. Remember, your path to wellness is a continuous journey of learning and adapting. Stay curious, and keep informed.

Appendix B:
Recipes for a Healthier Lifestyle

The journey to a healthier lifestyle is greatly enhanced when we bring delicious and nutritious meals to our table. This appendix provides a selection of recipes that not only avoid harmful sugars and processed oils but also celebrate the joy of cooking with whole, nourishing ingredients. These recipes are designed to be accessible to all skill levels and can be enjoyed by everyone from health-conscious individuals to families aiming to improve their overall well-being.

1. Hearty Quinoa Salad

This salad is a powerhouse of nutrition, loaded with fiber, protein, and antioxidants. It's perfect for lunch or as a light dinner.

- 1 cup quinoa, rinsed
- 2 cups water or vegetable broth
- 1 cup cherry tomatoes, halved
- 1 cucumber, diced
- 1/4 red onion, finely chopped
- 1/2 cup feta cheese, crumbled (optional)
- 1/4 cup fresh parsley, chopped
- 2 tablespoons olive oil
- 1 tablespoon lemon juice

- Salt and pepper to taste

Instructions:

1. In a medium saucepan, combine quinoa and water (or broth). Bring to a boil, then reduce heat and simmer for 15-20 minutes, or until quinoa is tender and water is absorbed. Let it cool.

2. In a large bowl, mix the cooked quinoa, cherry tomatoes, cucumber, red onion, feta cheese, and parsley.

3. In a small bowl, whisk together olive oil, lemon juice, salt, and pepper. Pour over quinoa mixture and toss to coat.

4. Serve immediately or refrigerate for up to two days.

2. Baked Salmon with Avocado Salsa

This dish provides a heart-healthy serving of omega-3 fatty acids, paired with a zesty avocado salsa for a refreshing and satisfying meal.

- 4 salmon fillets
- 2 tablespoons olive oil
- 1 teaspoon paprika
- Salt and pepper to taste
- 1 avocado, diced
- 1 small tomato, diced
- 1/4 red onion, finely chopped
- 1 jalapeño, seeded and minced (optional)
- 2 tablespoons cilantro, chopped
- 1 tablespoon lime juice

Instructions:

1. Preheat your oven to 375°F (190°C). Line a baking sheet with parchment paper.

2. Place salmon fillets on the prepared baking sheet. Drizzle with olive oil and sprinkle with paprika, salt, and pepper.

3. Bake for 15-20 minutes, or until the salmon is cooked through and flakes easily with a fork.

4. While the salmon is baking, prepare the avocado salsa by mixing the diced avocado, tomato, red onion, jalapeño (if using), cilantro, and lime juice in a medium bowl. Season with salt and pepper.

5. Serve the baked salmon topped with the fresh avocado salsa.

3. Flourless Banana Pancakes

These pancakes are a delightful way to start your day, free from refined sugars and full of natural sweetness from bananas.

- 2 ripe bananas, mashed
- 2 eggs
- 1/2 teaspoon vanilla extract
- 1/2 teaspoon baking powder
- Pinch of salt
- 1/4 teaspoon ground cinnamon (optional)
- Cooking spray or a small amount of coconut oil for the pan

Instructions:

1. In a medium bowl, whisk together mashed bananas, eggs, vanilla extract, baking powder, salt, and cinnamon (if using).

2. Heat a non-stick skillet over medium heat and lightly grease with cooking spray or coconut oil.

3. Pour small amounts of batter (around 2 tablespoons) onto the skillet to form pancakes. Cook until bubbles form on the surface, then flip and cook until both sides are golden brown.

4. Serve warm, topped with fresh fruit, a drizzle of honey, or a dollop of Greek yogurt.

These recipes are just a starting point. Experiment with whole foods and natural ingredients to create meals that not only nourish your body but also bring joy to your table. Eating healthier doesn't have to be restrictive; it can be an exciting journey of discovery and flavor.

References:

(Perlmutter, 2021)

(Fung, 2016)

(Teicholz, 2014)

Glossary of Terms

Understanding the various terms related to sugar and processed oils can empower you to make informed choices about your diet and health. This glossary explains key concepts and terminology used throughout the book.

Added Sugars

Sugars and syrups that are added to foods or beverages during processing or preparation. They do not include naturally occurring sugars found in milk and fruits (Johnson et al., 2009).

Cardiovascular Health

The health of the heart and blood vessels. Good cardiovascular health is crucial for overall well-being and can be negatively affected by processed oils and excessive sugar intake (Mozaffarian et al., 2010).

Chronic Diseases

Long-lasting health conditions that can be controlled but often not cured. Conditions such as diabetes, heart disease, and obesity are linked to poor diet choices, including high consumption of sugar and unhealthy fats (World Health Organization, 2021).

Fats

Essential macro-nutrients required for various bodily functions. They are categorized into saturated, monounsaturated, and polyunsaturated fats, all of which have distinct roles and impacts on health (Harvard T.H. Chan School of Public Health, n.d.).

Glucose

A simple sugar that is an important energy source in living organisms and is a component of many carbohydrates. Excess glucose in the diet can lead to health issues like diabetes (American Diabetes Association, n.d.).

High-Fructose Corn Syrup (HFCS)

A sweetener made from corn starch that has been processed to convert glucose into fructose. HFCS is commonly found in soft drinks and processed foods and is linked to obesity and metabolic disorders (Bray et al., 2004).

Hydrogenated Oils

Oils that have been chemically altered by adding hydrogen to increase shelf life and stability. This process creates trans fats, which are harmful to cardiovascular health (Kummerow, 2013).

Monounsaturated Fats

Fats found in foods like avocados, nuts, and olive oil. They are considered heart-healthy and beneficial when consumed in moderation (Harvard T.H. Chan School of Public Health, n.d.).

Natural Sugars

Sugars found naturally in whole foods such as fruits, vegetables, and dairy products. Unlike added sugars, natural sugars come with essential nutrients and fiber (Mann, 2014).

Omega-3 Fatty Acids

A type of polyunsaturated fat that is beneficial for heart health and found in fish, flaxseeds, and walnuts (Swanson et al., 2012).

Polyunsaturated Fats

Found in plant-based oils and fish, these fats include essential omega-3 and omega-6 fatty acids, which are crucial for brain function and cell growth (Harvard T.H. Chan School of Public Health, n.d.).

Processed Oils

Oils that have undergone chemical treatments and refining. These oils are often high in trans fats and can contribute to inflammation and chronic disease (Mozaffarian et al., 2010).

Saturated Fats

Fats that are solid at room temperature and found in animal products and some plants. While necessary in small amounts, excessive consumption can lead to health issues (Hu et al., 2001).

Trans Fats

Unhealthy fats formed during the hydrogenation of oils. Found in some margarines, snack foods, and fried foods, they are particularly harmful to heart health (Kummerow, 2013).

Whole Foods

Foods that are unprocessed or minimally processed, retaining their natural nutrients and fiber. Examples include fruits, vegetables, whole grains, and unprocessed meats (Pollan, 2009).

Vegetable Oils

Oils extracted from seeds or parts of fruits. While some, like olive oil, are healthy, others, like soybean oil, can be heavily processed and detrimental to health (Mozaffarian et al., 2010).

References

1. Huth, P. J., DiRienzo, D. B., & Miller, G. D. (2006). Major scientific advances with dairy foods in nutrition and health. Journal of Dairy Science, 89(4), 1207-1221.

2. Liu, S., Willett, W. C., Manson, J. E., Hu, F. B., Rosner, B., & Colditz, G. (2000). Relation between changes in intakes of dietary fiber and grain products and changes in weight and development of obesity among middle-aged women. American Journal of Clinical Nutrition, 78(5), 920-927.

3. Phillips, S. M., & Van Loon, L. J. C. (2011). Dietary protein for athletes: from requirements to optimum adaptation. Journal of Sports Sciences, 29(sup1), S29-S38.

4. Slavin, J. L. (2005). Dietary fiber and body weight. Nutrition, 21(3), 411–418.

5. Tipton, K. D., & Wolfe, R. R. (2001). Exercise, protein metabolism, and muscle growth. International Journal of Sport Nutrition and Exercise Metabolism, 11(1), 109-132.

6. (Innis, 2007) Innis, S. M. (2007). Dietary (n-3) fatty acids and brain development. The Journal of Nutrition, 137(4), 855-859.

7. (Mensink, 2001) Mensink, R. P. (2001). Effects of monounsaturated fatty acids on cardiovascular risk factors and outcomes in humans. Lipids, 36(11), 1138-1152.

8. (Mozaffarian et al., 2006) Mozaffarian, D., Katan, M. B., Ascherio, A., Stampfer, M. J., & Willett, W. C. (2006). Trans

fatty acids and cardiovascular disease. New England Journal of Medicine, 354(15), 1601-1613.

9. Astrup, A., Magkos, F., Bier, D. M., Brenna, J. T., de Oliveira Otto, M. C., Hill, J. O., ... & Krauss, R. M. (2021). Dietary fats and cardiovascular disease: A review of the evidence. American Journal of Clinical Nutrition, 113(4), 1009-1024.

10. Malik, V. S., Popkin, B. M., Bray, G. A., Després, J. P., Willett, W. C., & Hu, F. B. (2010). Sugar-sweetened beverages and risk of metabolic syndrome and type 2 diabetes: a meta-analysis. The Lancet, 375(9718), 736-741.

11. Moss, M. (2013). Salt Sugar Fat: How the Food Giants Hooked Us. Random House.

12. Seidelmann, S. B., Claggett, B., Cheng, S., Henglin, M., Shah, A., Steffen, L. M., ... & Solomon, S. D. (2018). Dietary carbohydrate intake and mortality: a prospective cohort study and meta-analysis. Lancet Public Health, 3(9), e419-e428.

13. Taubes, G. (2007). Good Calories, Bad Calories. Knopf.

14. Teicholz, N. (2014). The Big Fat Surprise: Why Butter, Meat, and Cheese Belong in a Healthy Diet. Simon & Schuster.

15. Marketing to the Masses: Seeing Past the Health Hype taps into the heart of consumer decision-making. It explores how marketing tactics can mislead even the most discerning buyers. With its combination of scientific insight, motivational drive, and practical advice, this section empowers you to see beyond the health claims plastered all over food packaging.

16. (AHA, 2020). American Heart Association. "Added Sugars." Retrieved from https://www.heart.org/en/healthy-living/healthy-eating/eat-smart/sugar/added-sugars

17. (CDC, 2021). Centers for Disease Control and Prevention. "Sugar and Your Health." Retrieved from https://www.cdc.gov/nutrition/data-statistics/sugar.html

18. (DiNicolantonio, J. J., O'Keefe, J. H., & Wilson, W. L., 2018). "Sugar Addiction: Is It Real? A Narrative Review." British Journal of Sports Medicine, 52(10), 910-913.

19. (Hu, F. B., 2013). "Resolved: There Is Sufficient Scientific Evidence That Decreasing Sugar-Sweetened Beverage Consumption Will Reduce the Prevalence of Obesity and Obesity-Related Diseases." Obesity Reviews, 14(8), 606-619.

20. (Johnson, R. K., Appel, L. J., Brands, M., Howard, B. V., Lefevre, M., Lustig, R. H., Sacks, F. M., Steffen, L. M., & Wylie-Rosett, J., 2009). "Dietary Sugars Intake and Cardiovascular Health: A Scientific Statement From the American Heart Association." Circulation, 120(11), 1011-1020.

21. (Ludwig, D. S., 2002). The Glycemic Index: Physiological Mechanisms Relating to Obesity, Diabetes, and Cardiovascular Disease. JAMA, 287(18), 2414-2423. doi:10.1001/jama.287.18.2414

22. (Lustig, R. H., 2012). "Fat Chance: Beating the Odds Against Sugar, Processed Food, Obesity, and Disease."

23. (Micha, R., Peñalvo, J. L., Cudhea, F., Imamura, F., Rehm, C. D., & Mozaffarian, D., 2017). Association Between Dietary Factors and Mortality From Heart Disease, Stroke, and Type 2 Diabetes in the United States. JAMA, 317(9), 912-924. doi:10.1001/jama.2017.0947

24. (Mozaffarian, D., Angell, S. Y., Lang, T., Hickey, T., 2018). The Plight of Fruits and Vegetables: A Global Call for Policy Action. Global Obesity, 24(3), 27-36. doi:10.1038/s41893-020-0492-7

25.   (Stanhope, K. L., 2016). "Sugar Consumption, Metabolic Disease and Obesity: The State of the Controversy." Critical Reviews in Clinical Laboratory Sciences, 53(1), 52-67.

26.   - Ghosh, S., et al. (2021). The history, status, and future perspectives on and the past, present, and future of margarine and shortening. Food Research International, 141, 110188. https://doi.org/10.1016/j.foodres.2021.110188

27.   - Harvard T.H. Chan School of Public Health. (n.d.). Types of fat.   Retrieved   from https://www.hsph.harvard.edu/nutritionsource/what-should-you-eat/fats-and-cholesterol/types-of-fat/

28.   - Keys, A., et al. (1984). Serum cholesterol response to changes in the diet: IV. Particular saturated fatty acids in the diet. Metabolism, 33(11), 1016-1020. https://doi.org/10.1016/0026-0495(84)90022-1

29.   - Mozaffarian, D., et al. (2006). Trans fatty acids and cardiovascular disease. New England Journal of Medicine, 354(15), 1601-1613. https://doi.org/10.1056/NEJMra054035

30.   - Nestle, M. (2013). Food politics: How the food industry influences nutrition and health. University of California Press.

31.   Aggarwal, B. B., & Sung, B. (2009). Pharmacological basis for the role of curcumin in chronic diseases: An age-old spice with modern targets. Trends in Pharmacological Sciences, 30(2), 85-94.

32.   Al-Farsi, M. A., & Lee, C. Y. (2008). Nutritional and functional properties of dates: a review. Critical Reviews in Food Science and Nutrition, 48(10), 877-887.

33. Arumughan, M., Subash, W., & Sindhu, R.K. (2009). Coconut sap sugar and its chemistry. Plant Foods for Human Nutrition, 64(2), 105-113.

34. Astrup, A., Dyerberg, J., Elwood, P., et al. (2011). The role of reducing intakes of saturated fat in the prevention of cardiovascular disease: where does the evidence stand in 2010?. The American Journal of Clinical Nutrition, 93(4), 684-686.

35. Barrett, C. (2002). Honey in Ancient Egypt. Cambridge University Press.

36. Bhupathiraju, S. N., & Hu, F. B. (2016). Epidemiology of obesity and diabetes and their cardiovascular complications. Circulation Research, 118(11), 1723-1735.

37. Bogdanov, S., Jurendic T., Sieber R., & Gallmann P. (2008). Honey for nutrition and health: a review. Journal of the American College of Nutrition, 27(6), 677-689.

38. Bray, G. A., Nielsen, S. J., & Popkin, B. M. (2004). Consumption of high-fructose corn syrup in beverages may play a role in the epidemic of obesity. *American Journal of Clinical Nutrition*, 79(4), 537-543.

39. Bray, G. A., Nielsen, S. J., & Popkin, B. M. (2004). Consumption of high-fructose corn syrup in beverages may play a role in the epidemic of obesity. American Journal of Clinical Nutrition, 79(4), 537-543.

40. Calder, P. C. (2008). Polyunsaturated fatty acids, inflammatory processes and inflammatory bowel diseases. Molecular Nutrition & Food Research, 52(8), 885-897.

41. Calder, P. C. (2015). Omega-3 polyunsaturated fatty acids and inflammatory processes: Nutrition or pharmacology?. British Journal of Clinical Pharmacology, 75(3), 675-685.

42. Chatsudthipong, V., & Muanprasat, C. (2009). Stevioside and related compounds: Therapeutic benefits beyond sweetness. Pharmacology & Therapeutics, 121(1), 41-54.

43. Dashti, H. S., Smith, C. E., Lee, Y., & McKeown, N. M. (2017). Dietary patterns and cardiovascular disease risk. Current Opinion in Lipidology, 28(4), 318–322.

44. DeBose, R., Johnson, J., & Wu, C. (2020). "Nutritional Importance of Fats in Childhood Development". Journal of Pediatric Health, 112(3), 56-67.

45. Devaraj, S., Wang-Polagruto, J., Polagruto, J., Keen, C. L., & Jialal, I. (2008). High-fat, energy-dense, fast-food–style breakfast results in an increase in oxidative stress in metabolic syndrome. Metabolism, 57(6), 867-870.

46. Downs, S. M., Thow, A. M., & Leeder, S. R. (2013). The effectiveness of policies for reducing dietary trans fat: a systematic review of the evidence. *Bulletin of the World Health Organization, 91*(4), 262-269H.

47. Eaton, S. B. (2019). The evolutionary context of human diet and health. Nutrition in Clinical Practice, 21(1), 603-606.

48. Estruch, R., Ros, E., Salas-Salvadó, J., Covas, M. I., Corella, D., Arós, F., ... & Martínez-González, M. A. (2018). Primary prevention of cardiovascular disease with a Mediterranean diet supplemented with extra-virgin olive oil or nuts. The New England Journal of Medicine, 378(25), e34.

49. Gatenby, R. A., & Gillies, R. J. (2004). Why do cancers have high aerobic glycolysis? Nature Reviews Cancer, 4(11), 891-899.

50. Geurts, M., & Wendel-Vos, W. (2018). Supermarket layout and the impact on food choices. Appetite, 120, 401-407.

51. Goran, M. I., Ball, G. D., & Cruz, M. L. (2013). Obesity and risk of type 2 diabetes and cardiovascular diseases in children and adolescents. The Journal of Pediatrics, 152(5), 823-830.

52. Goyal, S. K., Samsher, & Goyal, R. K. (2010). Stevia (Stevia rebaudiana) a bio-sweetener: a review. International Journal of Food Sciences and Nutrition, 61(1), 1-10.

53. Gurr, M. I. (1992). Dietary Lipids and Health: Introduction. British Journal of Nutrition, 68(2), 1-22.

54. Han, J. C., Lawlor, D. A., & Kimm, S. Y. (2010). Childhood obesity. The Lancet, 375(9727), 1737-1748.

55. Hotamisligil, G. S. (2006). Inflammation and metabolic disorders. Nature, 444(7121), 860-867.

56. Hu, F. B. (2011). Globalization of diabetes: the role of diet, lifestyle, and genes. Diabetes Care, 34(6), 1249-1257.

57. Hu, F. B., & Malik, V. S. (2010). Sugar-sweetened beverages and risk of obesity and type 2 diabetes: Epidemiologic evidence. Physiology & Behavior, 100(1), 47-54. https://doi.org/10.1016/j.physbeh.2010.01.036

58. Hu, F. B., Manson, J. E., & Willett, W. C. (2001). Types of dietary fat and risk of coronary heart disease: A critical review. *Journal of the American College of Nutrition*, 20(1), 5-19.

59. Hu, F. B., Manson, J. E., & Willett, W. C. (2019). Types of dietary fat and risk of coronary heart disease: a critical review. *Journal of the American College of Nutrition*, *18*(3), 190-202.

60. Hu, F. B., Stampfer, M. J., Manson, J. E., Rimm, E. B., Colditz, G. A., Rosner, B. A., Hennekens, C. H., & Willett, W. C. (2001). Dietary fat intake and the risk of coronary heart disease

in women. *The New England Journal of Medicine, 337*(21), 1491-9.

61. Jacobson, M. F., & Willett, W. C. (2009). Coronary heart disease and dietary factors: Evidence-based food guides and policies. Nutrition Reviews, 67(III), S51-S56.

62. Jenkins, D. J., Kendall, C. W., & Marchie, A. (2015). Effect of altering glycemic index or load on postprandial glycemia and insulinemia in healthy young adults. *The American Journal of Clinical Nutrition*, *81*(5), 110-117.

63. Jenkins, D. J., Wolever, T. M., Taylor, R. H., Barker, H., Fielden, H., Baldwin, J. M., ... & Goff, D. V. (1981). Glycemic index of foods: a physiological basis for carbohydrate exchange. *American Journal of Clinical Nutrition*, 34(3), 362-366.

64. Jensen, J. D., Denver, S., Zanoli, R., Rasmussen, S., & Schepler, S. I. (2019). Consumer preferences for organic food and its impact on supply chains. British Food Journal, 121(7), 1744-1757.

65. Johnson, R. J., Segal, M. S., Sautin, Y., Nakagawa, T., Feig, D. I., Kang, D. H., ... & Tuttle, K. R. (2009). Potential role of sugar (fructose) in the epidemic of hypertension, obesity, and the metabolic syndrome, diabetes, kidney disease, and cardiovascular disease. American Journal of Clinical Nutrition, 86(4), 899-906.

66. Johnson, R. K., Appel, L. J., Brands, M., Howard, B. V., Lefevre, M., Lustig, R, H , ... & Wylie-Rosett, J. (2007). Dietary sugars intake and cardiovascular health: a scientific statement from the American Heart Association. Circulation, 120(11), 1011-1020.

67. Johnson, R. K., Appel, L. J., Brands, M., Howard, B. V., Lefevre, M., Lustig, R. H., ... & Wylie-Rosett, J. (2009). Dietary sugars intake and cardiovascular health: a scientific statement from the American Heart Association. Circulation, 120(11), 1011-1020.

68. Johnson, R. K., Appel, L. J., Brands, M., Howard, B. V., Lefevre, M., Lustig, R. H., ... & Wylie-Rosett, J. (2009). Dietary sugars intake and cardiovascular health: a scientific statement from the American Heart Association. Circulation, 120(11), 1011-1020.

69. Johnson, R. K., Appel, L. J., Brands, M., Howard, B. V., Lefevre, M., Lustig, R. H., Sacks, F., Steffen, L. M., & Wylie-Rosett, J. (2009). Dietary sugars intake and cardiovascular health: A scientific statement from the American Heart Association. Circulation, 120(11), 1011-1020.

70. Johnson, R. K., Appel, L. J., Brands, M., Howard, B. V., Lefevre, M., Lustig, R. H., … & Wylie-Rosett, J. (2009). Dietary sugars intake and cardiovascular health: a scientific statement from the American Heart Association. Circulation, 120(11), 1011-1020.

71. Johnson, S. W. (2007). The health benefits of honey as a natural sweetener. Journal of Nutrition Research, 26(3), 456-463.

72. Kanoski, S. E., & Davidson, T. L. (2011). Western diet consumption and cognitive impairment: Links to hippocampal dysfunction and obesity. Physiology & Behavior, 103(1), 59-68.

73. Katan, M. B., Zock, P. L., & Mensink, R. P. (1995). Dietary oils, serum lipoproteins, and coronary heart disease. *The American Journal of Clinical Nutrition, 61*(6), 1368S-1373S.

74. Kiple, K. F., & Ornelas, K. C. (2000). The Cambridge World History of Food. Cambridge University Press.

75. Kiple, K. F., & Ornelas, K. C. (2000). The Cambridge World History of Food. Cambridge University Press.

76. Libby, P. (2002). Inflammation in atherosclerosis. Nature, 420(6917), 868-874.

77. Libuda, L., Alexy, U., Remer, T., Stehle, P., & Kersting, M. (2008). Association between long-term consumption of soft drinks and variables of bone modeling and remodeling in a sample of healthy German children and adolescents. American Journal of Clinical Nutrition, 88(6), 1670-1677.

78. Livesey, G. (2009). Health potential of polyols as sugar replacers, with emphasis on low glycaemic properties. Nutrition Research Reviews, 16(2), 163-191.

79. Lohner, S., Toews, I., & Meerpohl, J. J. (2017). Health outcomes of non-nutritive sweeteners: analysis of the research landscape. Nutrition Journal, 16(1), 55.

80. Ludwig, D. S., & Ebbeling, C. B. (2018). The Carbohydrate-Insulin Model of Obesity: Beyond "Calories In, Calories Out". JAMA Internal Medicine, 178(8), 1098-1103.

81. Ludwig, D. S., & Nestle, M. (2008). Can the food industry play a constructive role in the obesity epidemic? JAMA, 300(15), 1808-1811.

82. Lustig, R. H. (2012). "Fat Chance: Beating the Odds Against Sugar, Processed Food, Obesity, and Disease." New York: Hudson Street Press.

83. Lustig, R. H. (2012). Fat Chance: Beating the Odds Against Sugar, Processed Food, Obesity, and Disease. Penguin Group USA.

84. Lustig, R. H. (2013). Fat Chance: Beating the Odds Against Sugar, Processed Food, Obesity, and Disease. New York, NY: Hudson Street Press.

85. Lustig, R. H. (2013). Fat chance: Beating the odds against sugar, processed food, obesity, and disease. New York: Hudson Street Press.

86. Lustig, R. H., Schmidt, L. A., & Brindis, C. D. (2012). Public health: The toxic truth about sugar. Nature, 482(7383), 27-29.

87. Lustig, R. H., Schmidt, L. A., & Brindis, C. D. (2012). Public health: The toxic truth about sugar. Nature, 482(7383), 27-29.

88. Malik, V. S., Popkin, B. M., Bray, G. A., Després, J. P., & Hu, F. B. (2010). Sugar-sweetened beverages, obesity, type 2 diabetes mellitus, and cardiovascular disease risk. Circulation, 121(11), 1356-1364.

89. Malik, V. S., Popkin, B. M., Bray, G. A., Després, J. P., & Willett, W. C. (2010). Sugar-sweetened beverages and risk of metabolic syndrome and type 2 diabetes: a meta-analysis. Diabetes Care, 33(11), 2477-2483.

90. Marketing tactics often leverage buzzwords like "organic," "natural," or "low-fat" to sway purchasing decisions. But these terms can be misleading. For instance, a product labeled "low-fat" may indeed have reduced fat content, but it could be teeming with added sugars, enhancing flavor at the cost of your health. Understanding these marketing ploys can equip you to make informed choices, cutting through the health hype and focusing on real nutritional value.

91. Mensink, R. P., & Katan, M. B. (1990). Effect of dietary trans fatty acids on high-density and low-density lipoprotein cholesterol levels in healthy subjects. *New England Journal of Medicine, 323*(7), 439-445.

92. Mensink, R. P., Zock, P. L., Kester, A. D., & Katan, M. B. (2003). Effects of dietary fatty acids and carbohydrates on the ratio of serum total to HDL cholesterol and on serum lipids and apolipoproteins: a meta-analysis of 60 controlled trials. The American Journal of Clinical Nutrition, 77(5), 1146-1155.

93. Micha, R., & Mozaffarian, D. (2010). Trans fatty acids: effects on metabolic syndrome, heart disease and diabetes. *Nature Reviews Endocrinology, 6*(6), 335-346.

94. Millichap, J. Gordon, & Yee, Michelle M. (2012). The Diet Factor in Attention-Deficit/Hyperactivity Disorder. Pediatrics, 129(2), 330-337.

95. Mintz, S. W. (1985). Sugar and Power: The Place of Sugar in Modern History. Viking.

96. Monaco, A., Capasso, L., & Conneally, C. (2019). Nutrition and functional foods. Critical Reviews in Food Science and Nutrition.

97. Monteiro, C. A., Cannon, G., Levy, R. B., Moubarac, J. C., Jaime, P., Martins, A., Canella, D., Louzada, M. L., & Parra, D. (2019). Ultra-processed foods: What they are and how to identify them. Public Health Nutrition, 22(5), 936-941.

98. Moss, M., & Gately, E. (2021). Hooked: Food, free will, and how the food giants exploit our addictions. New York: Random House.

99. Moynihan, Paula J., & Kelly, Sam P. (2014). Effect on Caries of Restricting Sugars Intake: Systematic Review to Inform WHO Guidelines. Journal of Dental Research, 93(1), 8-18.

100. Mozaffarian, D., & Clarke, R. (2009). Quantitative effects on cardiovascular risk factors and coronary heart disease risk of replacing partially hydrogenated vegetable oils with other fats and oils. European Journal of Clinical Nutrition, 63(S2), S22-S33.

101. Mozaffarian, D., Hao, T., Rimm, E. B., Willett, W. C., & Hu, F. B. (2019). Changes in Diet and Lifestyle and Long-Term Weight

Gain in Women and Men. New England Journal of Medicine, 364(25), 2392-2404.

102. Mozaffarian, D., Katan, M. B., Ascherio, A., Stampfer, M. J., & Willett, W. C. (2006). "Trans fatty acids and cardiovascular disease." New England Journal of Medicine, 354(15), 1601-1613.

103. Mozaffarian, D., Katan, M. B., Ascherio, A., Stampfer, M. J., & Willett, W. C. (2006). Trans fatty acids and cardiovascular disease. *New England Journal of Medicine, 354*(15), 1601-1613.

104. Mozaffarian, D., Katan, M. B., Ascherio, A., Stampfer, M. J., & Willett, W. C. (2006). Trans fatty acids and cardiovascular disease. New England Journal of Medicine, 354(15), 1601-1613. https://doi.org/10.1056/NEJMra054035

105. Mozaffarian, D., Katan, M. B., Ascherio, A., Stampfer, M. J., & Willett, W. C. (2006). Trans fatty acids and cardiovascular disease. New England Journal of Medicine, 354(15), 1601-1613.

106. Mozaffarian, D., Micha, R., & Wallace, S. (2010). Effects on coronary heart disease of increasing polyunsaturated fat in place of saturated fat: A systematic review and meta-analysis of randomized controlled trials. PLoS Medicine, 7(3), e1000252.

107. Mozaffarian, D., Wu, J. H., de Oliveira Otto, M. C., Sandesara, C. M., Dallas, L. G., Miyada, M. S., & Shearer, G. C. (2021). Omega-3 Fatty Acids and Cardiovascular Health. Arteriosclerosis, Thrombosis, and Vascular Biology, 32(3), 665-674.

108. Nestle, M. (2013). Food Politics: How the Food Industry Influences Nutrition and Health. Berkeley: University of California Press.

109. Noble, Emily E., & Kanoski, Scott E. (2016). Early life sugar consumption has long-term negative effects on memory function in male rats. Neuroscience, Nuroscience, 322, 34-45.

110. Nutritional Review. (2017). The health benefits of honey and maple syrup. Nutritional Review, 75(8), 624-636.

111. Pérez-Jiménez, F., & Ruano, J. (2001). Olive oil and cardiovascular health. The Olive Oil Source.

112. Reilly, John J., & Kelly, John. (2011). Long-term impact of overweight and obesity in childhood and adolescence on morbidity and premature mortality in adulthood: systematic review. International Journal of Obesity, 35 (7), 891-898.

113. Rettner, R. (2014). Omega-3 Fatty Acids Help Young Children Read Better: Study. Retrieved from https://www.livescience.com/43183-omega-3s-help-young-children-read-better.html

114. Rippe, J. M., & Angelopoulos, T. J. (2016). Sugars and Health Controversies: What Does the Science Say? Advances in Nutrition, 7(1), 14-26.

115. Rumessen, J. J., & Gudmand-Hoyer, E. (1986). Functional bowel disease: malabsorption and abdominal distress after ingestion of fructose, sorbitol, and fructose-sorbitol mixtures. *Gastroenterology*, 91(1), 58-67.

116. Santaren, I. D., Watkins, S. M., Liese, A. D., Wagenknecht, L. E., & Rewers, M. J. (2018). Serum sterols and risk of coronary artery disease: differences between whites and African Americans. Journal of Lipid Research, 59(12), 2251-2267.

117. Simopoulos, A. P. (2002). "Omega-3 fatty acids in the prevention-management of cardiovascular disease". Canadian Journal of Physiology and Pharmacology, 76(2), 353-359.

118. Simopoulos, A. P. (2002). The importance of the ratio of omega-6/omega-3 essential fatty acids. Biomedicine & Pharmacotherapy, 56(8), 365-379.

119. Simopoulos, A. P. (2016). Omega-3 fatty acids in inflammation and autoimmune diseases. Journal of the American College of Nutrition, 21(6), 495-505.

120. Siri-Tarino, P. W., Sun, Q., Hu, F. B., & Krauss, R. M. (2010). Meta-analysis of prospective cohort studies evaluating the association of saturated fat with cardiovascular disease. American Journal of Clinical Nutrition, 91(3), 535-546.

121. Slavin, J. L. (2005). Dietary fiber and body weight. Nutrition, 21(3), 411-418.

122. Smith, J. P., Brauer, M. P., & Davis, R. K. (2016). The impact of sugar and processed oils on chronic diseases. Annals of Nutritional Science, 42(1), 123-135.

123. St-Onge, M. P., & Bosarge, A. (2008). Weight-loss diet that includes consumption of medium-chain triacylglycerol oil leads to a greater rate of weight and fat mass loss than does olive oil. American Journal of Clinical Nutrition, 87(3), 621-626.

124. Stanhope, K. L., Schwarz, J. M., Keim, N. L., Griffen, S. C., Bremer, A. A., Graham, J. L., ... & Havel, P. J. (2009). Consuming fructose-sweetened, not glucose-sweetened, beverages increases visceral adiposity and lipids and decreases insulin sensitivity in overweight/obese humans. *Journal of Clinical Investigation*, 119(5), 1322-1334.

125. Stanhope, K. L., Schwarz, J. M., Keim, N. L., Griffen, S. C., Bremer, A. A., Graham, J. L., … & Havel, P. J. (2012). Effects of consuming fructose- or glucose-sweetened beverages for 10 weeks on fat deposition, lipid metabolism, and insulin

sensitivity in overweight/obese humans. Diabetes, 58(2), 234-242.

126. Stender, S., Dyerberg, J., & Astrup, A. (2006). High levels of industrially produced trans fat in popular fast foods. The New England journal of medicine, 354(15), 1650-1652. doi:10.1056/NEJMc062990

127. Swithers, S. E. (2013). Artificial sweeteners produce the counterintuitive effect of inducing metabolic derangements. Trends in Endocrinology & Metabolism, 24(9), 431-441.

128. Taras, H. (2005). Nutrition and student performance at school. Journal of School Health, 75(6), 199-213.

129. Te Morenga, L., Mallard, S., & Mann, J. (2013). "Dietary sugars and body weight: Systematic review and meta-analyses of randomized controlled trials and cohort studies." BMJ, 346, e7492.

130. Te Morenga, L., Mallard, S., & Mann, J. (2013). Dietary sugars and body weight: Systematic review and meta-analyses of randomized controlled trials and cohort studies. BMJ, 346, e7492.

131. Teicholz, N. (2014). The Big Fat Surprise: Why Butter, Meat and Cheese Belong in a Healthy Diet. Simon & Schuster.

132. Teicholz, N. (2014). The Big Fat Surprise: Why Butter, Meat, and Cheese Belong in a Healthy Diet. Simon & Schuster.

133. The modern consumer is bombarded with a barrage of health claims. Every product on the shelf seems to boast about being the healthiest, the most natural, or the most beneficial for your well-being. But here's the catch: Not all these claims are as straightforward as they appear. The food industry employs an arsenal of marketing strategies designed to sell their products,

often at the expense of your health (Nestle, 2013). Their goal is to make foods seem healthier than they are, masking the hidden sugars and unhealthy fats lurking within.

134. U.S. Department of Agriculture (USDA). (2021). Added sugars: definition and practical guides for intake. Nutrition and Health.

135. White, J. S. (2008). Straight talk about high-fructose corn syrup: what it is and what it ain't. *American Journal of Clinical Nutrition*, 88(6), 1716S-1721S.

136. Willett, W., et al. (2019). Dietary fats and prevention of cardiovascular disease. Journal of the American College of Cardiology, 73(16), 2026-2041.

137. Willett, W.C., Sacks, F., Trichopoulou, A., Drescher, G., Ferro-Luzzi, A., Helsing, E., & Trichopoulos, D. (1995). Mediterranean diet pyramid: A cultural model for healthy eating. American Journal of Clinical Nutrition, 61(6 Suppl), 1402S-1406S.

138. Wolraich, M. L., Lindgren, S. D., Stumbo, P. J., Stegink, L. D., Appelbaum, M. I., & Kiritsy, M. C. (1994). "Effects of diets high in sucrose or aspartame on the behavior and cognitive performance of children." New England Journal of Medicine, 330(5), 301-307.

139. World Health Organization. (2021). Noncommunicable diseases. Retrieved from https://www.who.int/news-room/fact-sheets/detail/noncommunicable-diseases

140. Yudkin, J. (1972). Pure, White, and Deadly. Pengin Adult HC/TR.

www.ingramcontent.com/pod-product-compliance
Lightning Source LLC
Chambersburg PA
CBHW022101020426
42335CB00012B/780